IMPROVE YOUR

MEMRY

EVERY DAY

D1315215

IMPROVE YOUR MEMORY EVERY DAY

ROBERT ALLEN

COLLINS & BROWN

This edition published in the United Kingdom in 2015 by
Collins & Brown
1 Gower Street
London
WC1E 6HD

An imprint of Pavilion Books Company Ltd

Copyright © Collins & Brown 2004, 2015
Text copyright © Robert Allen 2004, 2015

The moral right of the author has been asserted.

Distributed in the United States and Canada by
Sterling Publishing Co, Inc.
387 Park Avenue South
New York
NY 10016–8810

All rights reserved. No part of this publication may be copied, displayed, extracted,
reproduced, utilized, stored in a retrieval system or transmitted in any form or by any
means, electronic, mechanical or otherwise including but not limited to photocopying,
recording, or scanning without the prior written permission of the publishers.

ISBN 978-1-910231-36-4

A CIP catalogue record for this book is available from the British Library.

10 9 8 7 6 5 4 3 2 1

Reproduction by Colour Depth Ltd, UK
Printed and bound by Times Offset (M) Sdn Bhd, Malaysia

This book can be ordered direct from the publisher at www.pavilionbooks.com

Cover illustrations: Shutterstock
Illustrated by Jane Smith (illustration on pages 24-25 by Kang Chen)
Diagrams by Jon Morgan

Contents

Introduction: thanks for the memory

Compulsory introduction – this means YOU!

Memory is like a muscle – the more you work it, the stronger it gets.

Most introductions just fill up a bit of space at the front of the book. This one tells you important stuff about memory, how to improve it and how this book works. So read it. Please.

My aim is simple: to give you a powerful memory in the shortest time possible. The good news? You can make significant improvements to your memory in as little as a day. You may think that claim sounds overconfident or even fraudulent but it's the truth. There are a few simple tricks that you can learn today that will immediately improve your memory greatly.

What is memory?

Memory may seem like a handy tool that helps you find where you left your car keys but, if you think just a little deeper, it is far more important than that.

Memory is who you are

The fact that from moment to moment you have a stable sense of identity and that, as far as you are aware, the person who went to bed last night is the same person who woke up in the same bed this morning, is what allows you to be a person. Without memory, this would simply not be possible. This applies not just to individuals but to whole societies. Because we remember, we are able to hold opinions about other people, places, things, events. Imagine what life would be like without this faculty!

As we go through life we accumulate more and more memories. We call this experience and it is very valuable. It means that we often don't have to solve a problem or guess what is going to happen next because, thanks to experience, we have been there many times before and know just how

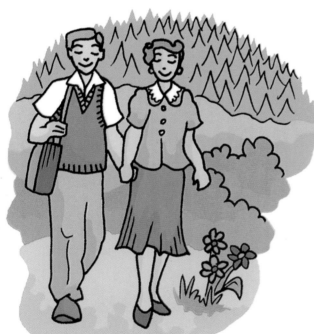

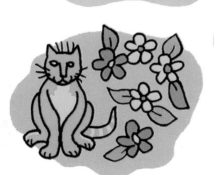

things are likely to pan out. When they were little, my children were convinced that I had some magic power that enabled me to predict what would happen next in a TV programme. It didn't occur to them that I had seen so many similar shows in the past that there was little room for the programme makers to fool me. Experience is also the reason why young people, whose intelligence is quick and active, are often out-thought by older people. The oldies may think more slowly but, for much of the time, they don't have to think at all because their experience tells them what's likely to be the answer. Youngsters score better where the problem is of a type not seen before. Which is one reason why kids outshine their elders when it comes to new technology.

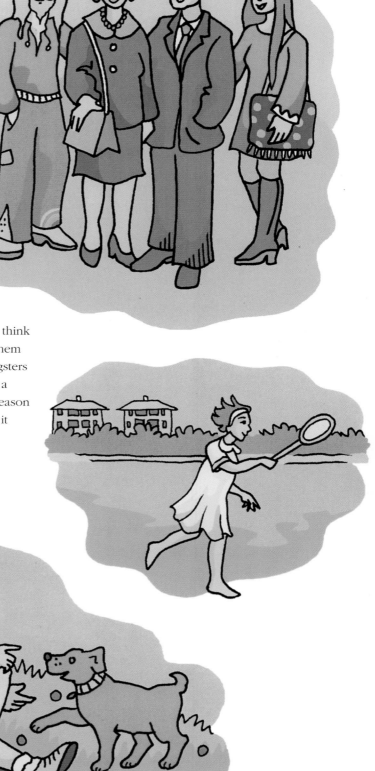

Remembering Rosebud

Memory is absolutely NOT a computer-style record of the past. It is quirky in the extreme. We often remember things for no obvious reason and forget things we would really like to remember. Do you recall Rosebud in the movie *Citizen Kane*? Why, of all the things he could have said, did Kane die with the word 'Rosebud' on his lips? That, of course, is the puzzle of the entire film and even though we finally discover that it was the name of the toboggan he owned as a kid, there are endless arguments over why he said it as he lay dying.

One of the reasons memory is so valuable is precisely because it is not mechanical. Our minds work to improve our memories. Without any conscious help from us, they add a gloss to our recollections. They can also blot out memories that are so unpalatable that the mind would rather not recall them at all. But memory can do so much more than

If you start today and practise, practise, practise, soon your memory will be as retentive as flypaper (though what gets stuck to it will, with luck, be more useful).

this. It can produce, at just the right moment, a piece of information you had long forgotten you possessed. If you have ever worked on a creative project you will

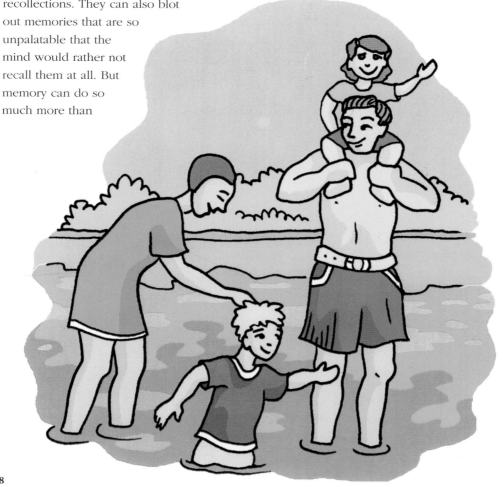

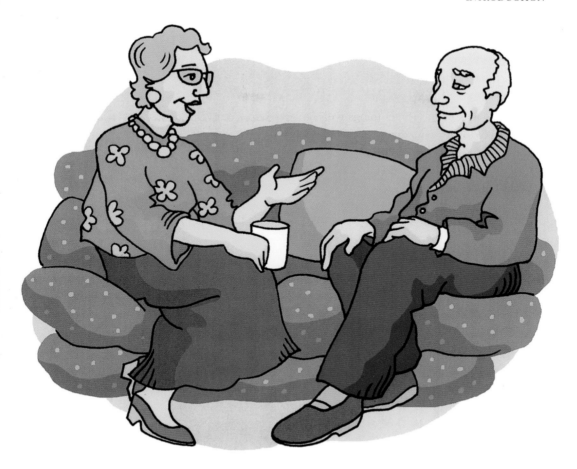

know only too well how your memory can throw up, quite unbidden, the most amazing treasures that you didn't know you still owned. So, far from being a cold, dead record of things past, the memory is like an Aladdin's cave crammed with the most amazing treasures.

We can never have free access to the cave of our memories but we can, with just a little practice, train ourselves to find things that we have deposited in the cave. This is a very valuable skill and it is one that you can acquire with very little effort if you just work on the exercises in this book.

Memory is a crazy woman that hoards coloured rags and throws away food.

Austin O'Malley

It doesn't matter who my father was; it matters who I remember he was.

Anne Sexton

Nothing is more responsible for the good old days than a bad memory.

Robert Benchley

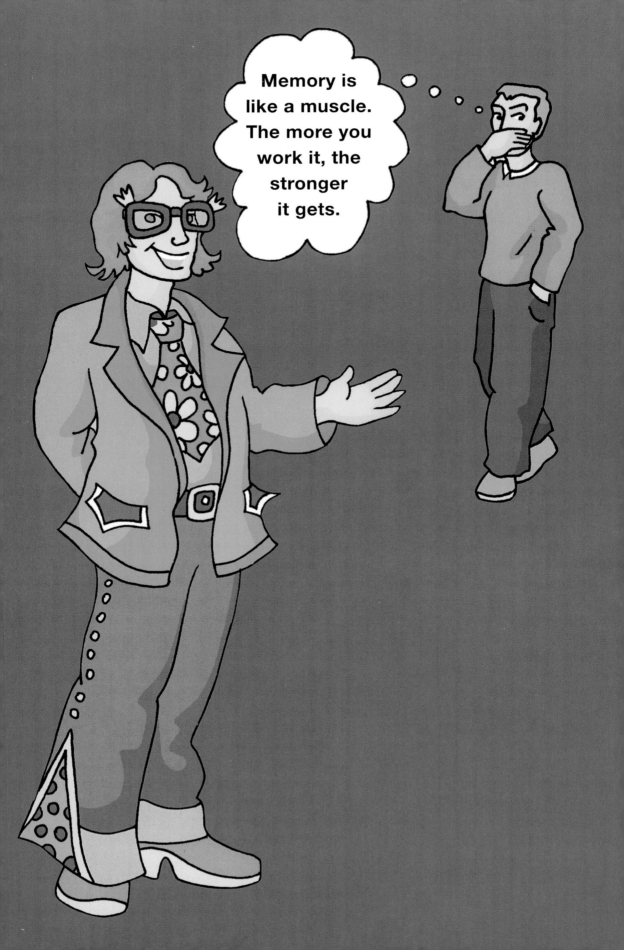

Memory Techniques

The first part of our course is devoted to finding out just how good your memory is now, and then teaching you how to improve it. You can learn a lot in a very short time, By the end of just one day of study, you will have at your disposal a variety of powerful memory tools that will last you a lifetime, But don't stop there! The more you use your new-found powers, the stronger they will become, Eventually, with regular practice, you will have a foolproof memory that will serve you well in all areas of your life.

You will have at your disposal a variety of powerful memory tools.

You can learn a lot in a very short time.

Become more efficient and professional.

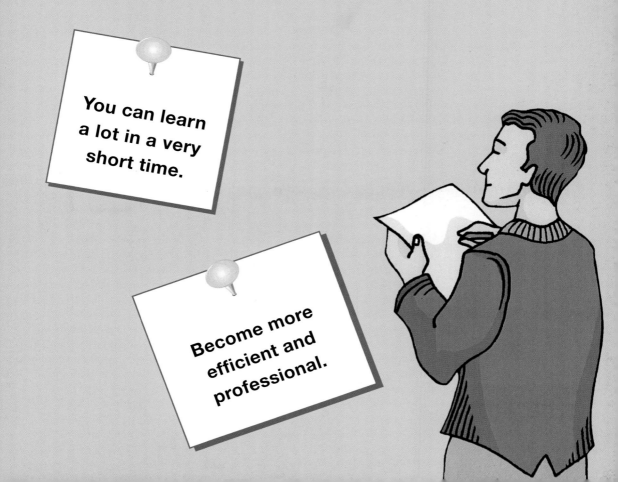

How do you learn?

There are three ways in which we learn: looking, listening and doing. Of these, most of us have a favourite that we tend to rely on, a second method we use as a back-up, and a third method that we feel less comfortable with. Some lucky people can use all three styles effectively and some unlucky people are completely deprived of one or more of them (for example, blind students can gain nothing from visual learning). The following test will tell you how you rate on each learning style. See 'What does it all mean?' (opposite), for a description of your personal learning style.

1   At a lecture, you may learn in several ways. Which is your favourite?
    a) Listening to the lecturer.
    b) Copying down notes from a whiteboard.
    c) Carrying out practical tasks based on what you learned in the lecture.

2   When you go to a movie, what do you remember best afterwards?
    a) The dialogue.
    b) The action sequences.
    c) The things you did: driving to the cinema, buying tickets and getting popcorn.

3   How would you learn to fix a flat bicycle tyre?
    a) Get a friend to describe how to do it.
    b) Buy a repair kit and read the instructions.
    c) Get to work with a spanner and figure it out for yourself.

4   If you wanted to learn the names of all the presidents of the USA, would you:
    a) Make up associations for each name (such as think of Lincoln as a car)?
    b) Look at portraits to help you remember their names?
    c) Get a set of pictures, cut them out, label them and put them in an album?

5   If you like a pop song, which of these activities would you enjoy most?
    a) Learning all the lyrics.
    b) Watching the video constantly.
    c) Trying to imitate the dance routine.

6   How well do you see things in your mind's eye?
    a) Poorly.
    b) Very well.
    c) Reasonably well.

7   When it comes to practical tasks using your hands, are you:
    a) Average?
    b) Excellent?
    c) Poor?

8   If someone reads you a story, do you:
    a) Remember it in great detail (parts of it word for word)?
    b) See a sort of home movie in your mind?
    c) Forget it quickly?

9   As a small child, which of these did you prefer?
    a) Reading.
    b) Drawing and painting.
    c) Playing with a shape sorter.

What does it all mean?

Listeners

If your answers are mostly 'a', you are a listener. You enjoy sounds, especially words, and you find they have powerful meanings for you. You are far more likely to remember and understand anything that you take in through your ears than information received through some other channel.

Lookers

If your answers are mostly 'b', you are a looker. You respond best to visual stimuli, which hold the most meaning for you. Anything you see will be easier to comprehend and retain than information from other sources.

Doers

If your answers are mostly 'c', you are a doer. You like to get your hands dirty (often quite literally). You learn best from practical experience – five minutes with your sleeves rolled up doing a practical job is, for you, a much more profound experience than several hours spent in a lecture theatre.

If you're lucky, you may have found that you answer equally well in more than one category. It is rare for anyone to learn exclusively in one style. Certainly, it is to your advantage to use all three learning styles wherever you can, because a combined attack is far more effective. If you find that you hardly use one style at all (looking, for example), you might have an undiagnosed problem in this area. An eye examination and a pair of glasses just might open up a whole new world to you.

10 If you moved to another town, how would you find your way around?
   a) Ask the locals for directions.
   b) Buy a map.
   c) Walk the streets until you became familiar with their layout.

11 Do you tend to remember best:
   a) The actual words people say to you?
   b) The way things look?
   c) Things that you do?

12 Which do you remember most vividly?
   a) Poems you learnt at school.
   b) What your childhood home looked like.
   c) How it felt to learn to swim.

13 When gardening, do you:
   a) Know the names of all the flowers and plants?
   b) Recognize plants but forget their names.
   c) Concentrate on practical tasks such as weeding and pruning?

14 Do you:
   a) Read a newspaper every day.
   b) Always make sure you see the news on IV
   c) Don't keep up with the news because you'd rather spend the time on something practical.

15 Which would cause you most distress?
   a) Having impaired hearing.
   b) Having impaired vision.
   c) Having impaired movement

Build your own powerhouse

Concentration is the powerhouse of memory. No matter how many tips and tricks you learn from this book, your memory will not reach its full potential unless you learn how to concentrate. This is not something that comes easily to most of us nor, in spite of its huge importance, is it something that we are taught at home or at school. When I was at school, the teachers would yell, 'Concentrate, boy!' but they might just as well have said, 'Levitate!' for all the good it did. I didn't know how to concentrate – not at will, anyway. Like most people, I could concentrate furiously on what interested me – a good book would do the trick but had trouble bending my mind to Latin case endings or quadratic equations.

When I was older and became interested in mind-training techniques, I discovered that concentration was considered a necessary skill in many Far Eastern cultures, and that there were techniques for teaching it. Here is one of them, which you might find useful. It is several millennia old, but none the worse for that:

☆ Light a candle and set it on a table in front of you.

☆ Stare at the candle for a couple of minutes. Try to remember every detail – the colour and texture of the wax, the appearance of the flame and the way it moves. Fix it all in your mind.

☆ Now close your eyes and try to retain the image of the candle in your mind's eye for as long as you can.

☆ Your first efforts will probably be pitiful. This exercise looks easy but isn't.

☆ Keep trying again and again. Eventually, you will be able to hold the image of the candle in your mind's eye for as long as you wish.

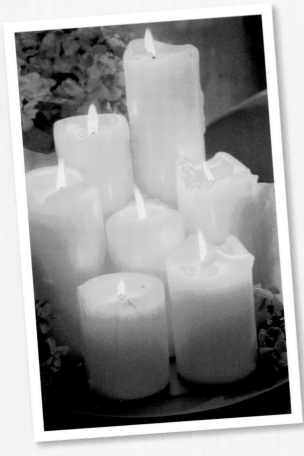

Concentration training

What other things must you do when you concentrate? One is to ,structure your time. Set aside a specific time for doing a particular task and try not to deviate from that. It is quite natural to sit down to a task, especially one that you don't really enjoy, and then think of something important you need to attend to. Then you fancy a coffee. Then you go to see if the post has arrived. Then the phone rings and you spend time chatting. Then, since you're already on the phone, you call a friend and waste some more time chatting. If you recognize this scenario, you not only need to practise concentration regularly, but also to structure your time. Make yourself a timetable and slot in all the tasks you hope to accomplish.

When you construct the timetable, bear in mind the way your day normally unfolds. Don't allot complicated tasks to times when you are usually disturbed. Remember that there are quiet times that often don't get used (early mornings, for example), which are really valuable if you need to work undisturbed.

If, as your work progresses, you find that your initial time estimates were faulty, you can correct them. That doesn't matter. But what does matter is that you stick to your task until it is accomplished and do NOT let yourself be distracted.

Incidentally, if you think I'm one of life's naturally ordered workers, who concentrates effortlessly, you'd be quite wrong. Everything I've written above is the product of bitter experience and oceans of wasted time. But now this section of the book is finished and I'm going for a coffee (after amending my timetable to show that it took me twenty minutes less than I'd planned).

Take a couple of minutes to consider whatever task is before you. Don't just rush into it, but consciously decide what methods you could use to complete it, and how long it should take. Once you have decided on the length of the session, stick to that decision and let nothing stop you.

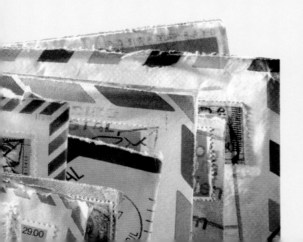

The truth is, a person's memory has no more sense than his conscience, and no appreciation whatever of values and proportions.
Mark Twain, *Eruption*

Body and mind

For your memory to work properly; you need to look after yourself. It's no good assuming that you can put your mind to work whenever you want and despite the way you have treated yourself. Remember that your body and your mind are one. In fact, your mind is all you will ever know. Anything that is outside your mind simply does not exist for you and never can exist, because the moment you are aware of it, it is part of your mind. Thus, even your body is only available to you as a mind object. So, looking after your mind and body is really; really important. Here are some things you need to bear in mind if you want to function properly. (None of what follows is very complicated. You've heard it all before. So, why aren't you doing it?)

Get enough sleep

This applies to everyone, but is particularly important to youngsters studying for exams. They are the ones who think that staying up until 3 a.m. every night chatting to their mates on the Internet is a really cool idea. It isn't. Sleep deprivation ruins concentration and reduces your ability to learn. It is also generally detrimental to your health.

Eat sensibly

A good diet is essential to mental and physical health. Junk food is called that for a reason. Try to eat lots of fresh fruit and vegetables. There is no specific brain food, but eating lots of pizzas, burgers and takeaways will do dreadful things not just to your memory but to your general health. One thing is very important: eat breakfast! Researchers have found that those who eat breakfast have better powers of recall than those who don't.

Get fresh air

Like concentration (see pages 14–15), breathing is something that we aren't taught. Of course we do it naturally; but there are ways to do it more efficiently. Make sure, when you work, that you have a window open. Keep the room at a comfortable but not excessive temperature. Learn to breathe properly (see 'Take a deep breath', opposite).

Get exercise

You don't have to live at the gym, but you do need a certain amount of exercise for your mind and body to function at maximum efficiency. Walking the dog (briskly) or mowing the lawn will do just as well, if you hate sports. But why not put in a little bit of extra effort

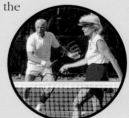

... little threads that hold life's patches of meaning together.
Mark Twain, Morals and Memory speech

TAKE A DEEP BREATH

Learn to breathe properly:

○ Sit quietly on a straight-backed chair.

○ Sit upright but don't strain (your muscles should be relaxed).

○ Imagine that there is a strong thread that connects the top of your head to the ceiling.

○ Tuck your chin in very slightly.

○ Close your eyes and breathe normally for a few minutes until your body and mind start to calm down naturally. Now comes the part that requires practice.

○ Very gently, draw the air down as far as you can. At first, you will only be able to get it down as far as your diaphragm. Surely that's enough? You can't go any lower, can you? Yes, actually you can. According to many Far Eastern schools of thought, there is an energy centre (called *hara* in Japanese and *Tan Tian* in Chinese) situated about 4 cm (½ inch) below the navel.

○ Try to draw the breath into this point – it is possible. All it takes is practice and, once you have learnt to breathe this way, you'll find that it has huge benefits for both mental and physical well-being.

and go for a long walk; or a swim? The dividends in both the long and the short-term are well worth the input.

Stuff to avoid

If you have never woken up in the morning unable to remember the events of the previous evening because you were a tad too enthusiastic with your drinking, I congratulate you. Most of us have done it at one time or another and you don't need me to tell you that it's a bad idea. If you want your memory to work well, booze is a very bad idea indeed, as are all drugs (including nicotine). An occasional indiscretion will produce a mere memory blip, but long-term abuse can mess up your mind in various unpleasant ways. Loss of memory will almost certainly be one of them.

The state of the art

How good is your memory right now? The following pages will seek to assess the current state of your memory with a series of tests that increase in difficulty. Just use whatever memory methods you normally use; it really doesn't matter if you do badly. The idea of this section is to show you just how much you can improve your memory by putting into practice the techniques taught later in the book.

SHORT-TERM MEMORY TASK 1

The 'Flurble' test

TIME: **3 minutes** LEVEL: **Easy**

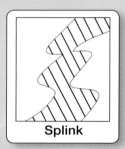
Splink

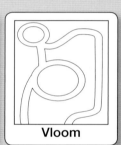
Vloom

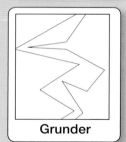
Grunder

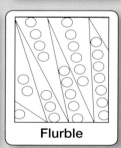
Flurble

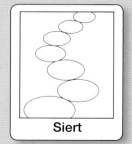
Siert

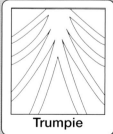
Trumpie

Instructions

1 Study the six pictures with strange names.
2 Spend three minutes memorizing them.
3 Now close the book, draw all six objects and write the correct names beneath them.
4 Check your answers against the original pictures.
5 Now spend a further five minutes – memorizing the original pictures.
6 Leave this exercise and then tomorrow, without further memorizing, try to draw and name what you can recall.

How did you do?

Although memory is always capable of improvement, if you were able to draw and name all six pictures on both occasions, your short-term memory is working well.

Retest: To test yourself further, go back to this task in, say, six weeks' time and see if the memory has become a long-term one.

Remember this!

Memory works best by association. Try to think of things that remind you of the shapes and names you are trying to memorize.

SHORT-TERM MEMORY TASK 2

It happened last Friday

TIME: **3 minutes** LEVEL: **Easy**

Here's another easy test of your short-term memory: All you have to do is read through the passage below. You can study it as hard as you like for three minutes, then cover the story and answer the questions:

Last Friday, Jim's wife, Sandra, asked him to go to the shops and buy some things ready for her parents' visit at the weekend. She needed a couple of pizza bases, some canned tomatoes, mozzarella and a couple of bottles of wine. She told him to go to Brown's because it was cheaper than Thompson's (and anyway Tommy Brown was her cousin). She told him to stop on the way back and get the car cleaned, and to pick up their twins, Mark and Michael, from school. Jim was almost home when he discovered that he'd forgotten the cheese, so he went back to town. This time he went to Thompson's, because it wasn't as far to drive. He also bought a bag of pretzels and some salted peanuts because he remembered that his father-in-law, Dick, liked them.

Questions

1 What is Jim's father-in-law called?
2 Which shop does his wife tell him to go to?
3 What does he forget on his first attempt?
4 Why does he go to Thompson's rather than Brown's on his second trip?
5 What are the names of Jim's twins?
6 Where is he supposed to pick them up?
7 What is Jim's wife called?
8 How many bottles of wine is Jim supposed to buy?
9 What canned goods does Jim's wife ask him to get?
10 What is he supposed to do with the car?
11 When are his wife's parents due to visit?
12 What is the connection between his wife and the owner of Brown's?
13 What sort of cheese does Jim forget to buy?
14 What does he buy specifically for his father-in-law?
15 On which day does the story take place?

SHORT-TERM MEMORY TASK 3
Kim's game
TIME: **3 minutes** LEVEL: **Medium**

Here's a more difficult task to test your visual memory. In Rudyard Kipling's book Kim, the young hero was trained in observation by being told to look at a tray full of objects and then, when the tray was removed, he had to remember as many of them as possible. Kim's game has long been a favourite at parties but it also has a serious role in memory training. There are 25 objects pictured on these pages. Your job is to look at them for three minutes and try to fix as many as possible in your mind. Then, with the book closed, write a list of what you can remember. If you don't get all the objects first time – and you'd have to have a very good memory to do that – you can have another go (and another) until you get the whole lot.

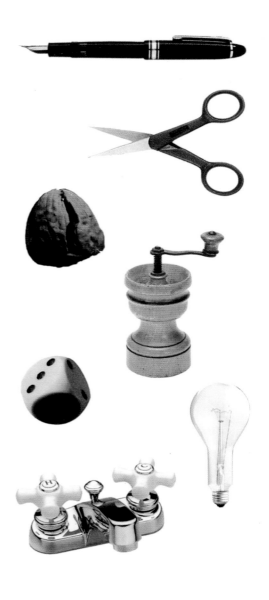

DON'T PANIC!
You won't be able to bring things to mind if you are in a panic. Give yourself time and work calmly. (If you're revising for a test or exam, start in plenty of time and don't try to do it all the night before.)

A diplomat is a man who always remembers a woman's birthday but never remembers her age.
Robert Frost

Can anybody remember when the times were not hard and money not scarce?
Ralph Waldo Emerson

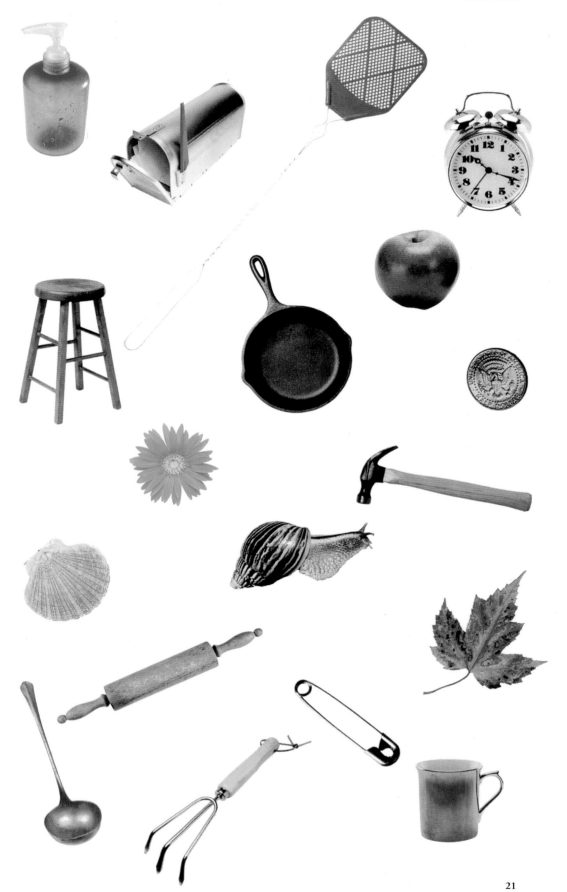

SHORT-TERM MEMORY TASK 4

Deceived by appearances

TIME: **3 minutes** LEVEL: **Medium**

This is one of those spot-the-difference games that will really test your visual memory. The picture on this page is the original and the one on the opposite page is the altered version. On this occasion, however, the game is played slightly differently from usual. You need to look at the left-hand image for three minutes and try to fix it in your mind, then cover it up and try to find fifteen differences in the right-hand picture.

The differences are all quite obvious. This is not a puzzle to test keen observation. All you need to do is fix the first picture firmly in your mind and then spot the major changes that have been made.

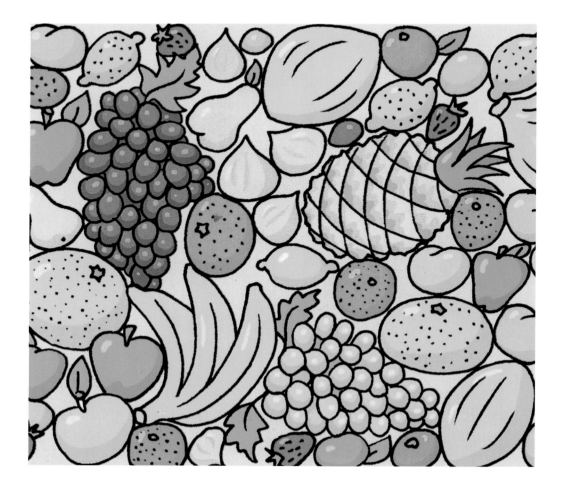

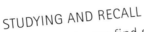

STUDYING AND RECALL

If, in spite of all the advice in this book, you find some facts just won't stick in your mind, take time to work out why. If they are too boring, use wild and wacky associations to make them more memorable. Really childish humour works wonders. But if you still get no result, consider why you cannot remember. Is your subconscious telling you that you're studying the wrong course?

Does the material that you're trying to remember have bad associations that you aren't acknowledging?

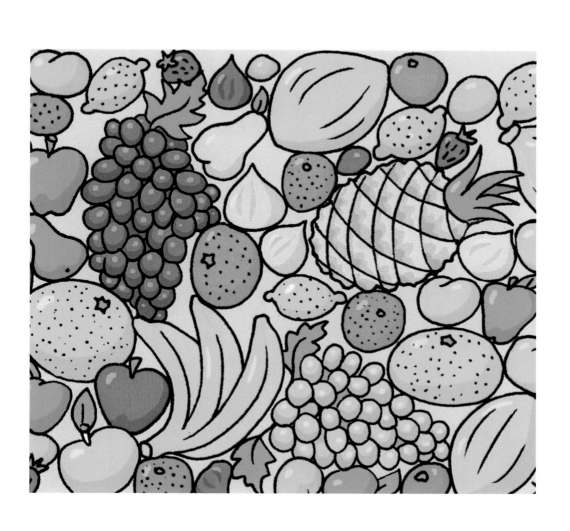

SHORT-TERM MEMORY TASK 5

Map memory

TIME: **10 minutes** LEVEL: **Medium**

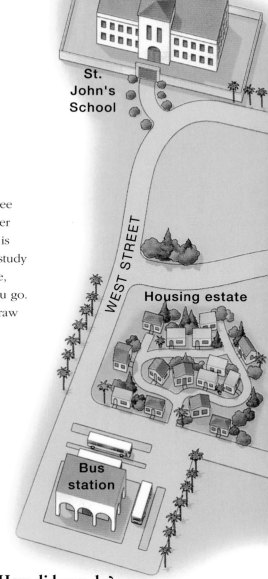

This test is about more than just visual memory (though that helps). The map contains a lot of diverse information (names, directions, objects). First, have a go at the whole map. Study it for three minutes, then cover the page with a piece of paper and try to answer the questions below. My guess is that you won't know many of the answers. Now study the map for a further seven minutes and, this time, draw the map and add the annotations to it as you go. Learn the main outlines first and, once you can draw these without error, start to add further details until you get the whole thing right.

1 What is the name of the church?
2 Which road runs from the church to West Street?
3 Which road connects Fen End and East Street?
4 What is situated in the south-west corner of the map?
5 What is situated north of the cemetery?
6 On which road is the pub situated?
7 What lies at the south end of Crossways?
8 In which road is the multi-storey car park?
9 What lies between West Street and Fen End?
10 What is situated at the extreme eastern edge of the town?
11 What is the town's main industrial concern?
12 What is the name of the school?
13 Which roads would you follow from the doctor's surgery to the cemetery?
14 What lies at the north end of West Street?
15 What is the quickest route from the doctor's surgery to the church?

How did you do?

If you really got all the questions right after only ten minutes' study, you are ready to become a professional poker player! The trick is to build up your memory bit by bit, filling in extra details as you go. Of course, if you were learning the layout of a real town, it would also make sense to get on your bike and ride around the streets so that you could learn them from personal experience.

If you had great difficulty with this task, don't worry, it is rather a tough one. Take your time and come back to this page later on. The good thing about memory is that

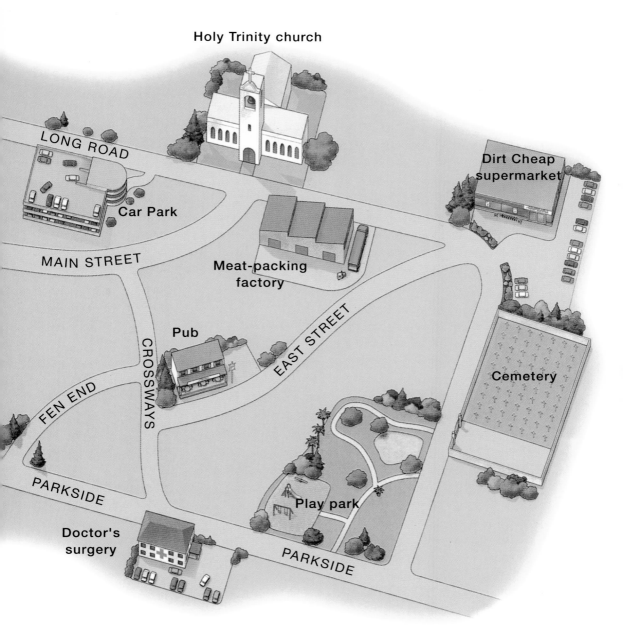

Holy Trinity church

LONG ROAD

Car Park

Dirt Cheap
supermarket

MAIN STREET

Meat-packing
factory

EAST STREET

Pub

Cemetery

CROSSWAYS

FEN END

PARKSIDE

Play park

Doctor's
surgery

PARKSIDE

practising a task like this will have a direct
effect on your ability to perform other
memory tasks. If you keep working at it,
you will soon be able to commit material to
memory quickly, accurately and painlessly

Remember this!

Learn to draw the town grid first, then
practise putting in the road names
followed by the buildings (working in a
clockwise direction).

The advantage of a bad memory is that one enjoys several times the same good things for the first time.

Friedrich Nietzsche

LONG-TERM MEMORY TASK

The good old days

Here's a test of your long-term memory. This is one area where older people tend to excel. Youngsters, whose brains are firing on all cylinders may, even so, find it harder to recall the distant past than their elders.

1 What was your grandmother's full name?

2 What was the address of the house you were born in?

3 What was your first cuddly toy called?

4 What was your favourite meal when you were a child?

5 What was your nickname at your first school?

6 What did your grandfather do for a living?

7 What did your grandfather look like?

8 Think of a present that you were given when you were under five years old.

9 Visualize the house you grew up in. What colour was the front door?

10 Who lived next door to you when you were little?

11 Can you picture your first day at school? What did you wear?

12 Who was your first teacher?

13 What was the naughtiest thing you did when you were little?

14 What is your earliest memory?

15 Who did you sit next to in school when you were eleven years old?

16 Which teacher did you really dislike intensely?

17 Can you still remember any poem, speech or reading you learnt by heart at school?

18 Who was the first person you had a crush on?

19 Who was the first person you dated?

20 Who first broke your heart?

21 Who was your best friend when you were eleven?

22 What is the first holiday you remember?

23 What are your earliest memories of Christmas (or other appropriate religious holiday)?

24 Describe a favourite toy.

25 When did you learn to ride a bike?

26 Who taught you to swim?

27 Who was your first real friend?

28 What was your favourite childhood game?

29 What was your favourite TV programme when you were five?

30 What was the first record you ever bought?

31 What was your nickname at school?

32 Do you have sharp pictures in your mind of events from the distant past?

33 Is there a smell that brings back particularly vivid memories for you?

34 What was your first pet called?

35 How many of your cuddly toys can you name?

36 Can you recall any of your birthday parties (below the age of eleven) in detail?

37 What was your favourite song when you were under five?

38 Did you have a gang when you were under eleven? Who else was in it?

39 Can you remember any near misses you had as a kid (such as a road accidents)?

40 What was your most serious childhood illness?

41 Do you have one favourite memory (from your whole life)?

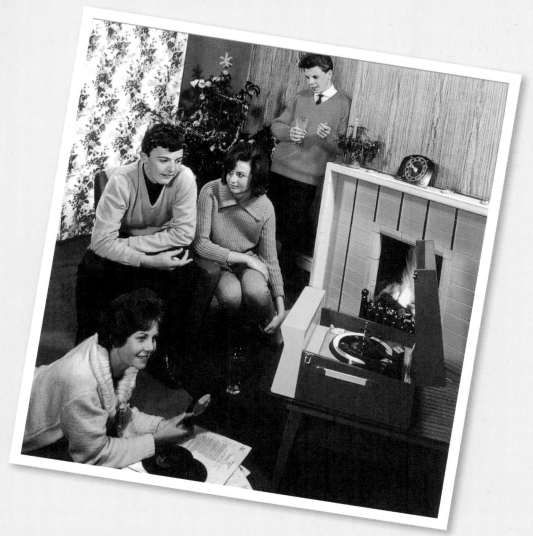

42 Is there one childhood friend you long to meet again?

43 Can you still remember stuff like science formulae that you learnt for exams?

44 Do you remember times long past more easily than recent events?

45 Can you remember where you were when you heard of the death of Diana, Princess of Wales?

How did you do?

The majority of people will have done well in this test and answered over 30 of the questions. What's more, it is likely that as you started to answer the questions, you were prompted to remember more and more. This mood of reverie may persist for quite some time. It might even prompt you to do things such as getting out old photos and souvenirs, phoning old acquaintances, or even trying to trace people you have lost touch with. Once you stimulate long-term memory, it becomes hugely powerful. You may well be startled at the amount of detail you store in your memory. I have found that just writing out the questions has released a powerful set of images from my childhood, and I can smell creosote on old wood heated in the sunshine – a smell I always associate with summer as a child.

How do we memorize?

Do you remember your first and last days at school? Almost certainly. Do you remember what you had for lunch a week ago? Almost certainly not. We only remember things that stick out in our memory.

I love that bit in cop films when the detective says to a suspect, 'What were you doing on 28 June at around six o'clock?' The suspect answers and then the detective trips him up with some well aimed information. Do you remember what you did last Thursday? Of course you don't. For something to be memorable, it must be made to stick out from the mass of completely forgettable detail that surrounds us. Think, for a moment, of all the information that passes in front of you every day. Think of all the cars, buses, trucks and people you see on your way to and from work. Can you remember any of them? No, normally not. But on the day there's an accident, you may well remember that it was a blue Mercedes driven by a guy in a red T-shirt that ended up on the wrong side of the road wrapped around a concrete lamp-post.

Memorization is simply a matter of making something stick in your mind. How do you make something stick? You use glue, of course! Memory is just another sort of glue. In fact, it is many sorts and, because you want to remember things for different amounts of time, you need different strengths of glue.

Here is a quick rundown of the methods we're going to use and a summary of what they are good for. We will look at each method in detail later.

Repetition

This is the weakest glue. Saying something over and over will make it stick in your mind for a very short while, then you'll forget it again. This is great for, say, a telephone number that you need just once.

Physical reminders

A physical reminder is something such as tying a knot in the corner of your handkerchief to help you remember. All little kids have done this at some time but, just because it's used by little kids doesn't mean that it won't work for you. It will. This method, however, works only briefly (which is all it was meant to do). It will remind you to pick up the kids from school, or take the car to the garage to be fixed, or pick up your dry-cleaning. Once it has accomplished the task, you get rid of it.

Ritual

This is a very weak glue that we use for a quick reminder. When she was too young to set her own alarm clock, my cousin had a system to ensure that she woke up at the right time. Before she got into bed, she'd turn around three times and each time she did it, she'd tap herself on the head and say, 'Six-thirty! Six-thirty! Six-thirty!' Then she'd jump into bed and yell, 'Goodnight world, see you at six-thirty!' It never failed. There are more complicated and useful ways to make ritual work for you (see page 42).

Narratives

I must be honest and admit that I never use this method. But that's no reason to leave it out of the book. I know people who swear by narratives. The method involves making up simple stories that connect a string of objects or facts to be remembered. For example, if you want to remember the telephone number 5231870, you could use a bit of imagination and turn it into, 'At five to three I ate seven cookies.' The trouble is that most information you'll want to memorize will need quite a leap of imagination to turn it into a narrative. I hope it works for you but, personally, there are techniques I like much better.

Association

For some crazy reason, it is easier to remember a thing if you associate it with another thing. For example, I could never remember the word 'cyclamen' (it's a plant, some people call it rabbit's ears). Then I noticed that the leaves look a bit like little wheels, so I called the plant 'cycling men' and now I never forget. Associations are good for remembering odd bits of simple information.

Mnemonics

A mnemonic is just a simple device to help you remember. It often, but not always, depends on the initial letters of words to be memorized, such as HOMES for the Great Lakes of America (Huron, Ontario, Michigan, Eyrie, Superior); or Richard Of York Gave Battle In Vain for the colours of the rainbow (Red, Orange, Yellow, Green, Blue, Indigo, Violet). Mnemonics are a strong glue and very useful. They help us remember a lot of stuff that is a drag to look up, and which we need to recall from time to time.

Rhythm and rhyme

We'll use rhythm and rhyme to cover both metre (as used in poetry) and music. You can use both of these to remember a wide variety of things. Beware! This is a very, very strong glue. Anything you remember this way will stay with you for life. When I was young, I memorized all my physics formulae to the tunes from Bizet's Carmen and now, forty years later, I still can't listen to that music without recalling stuff about amps and volts.

Visualization

This is also a strong glue, which is used for things such as remembering faces, diagrams and pictures. It can also be used in other very important ways that will be explained later (see pages 40–41).

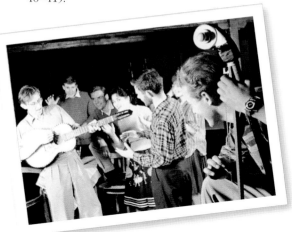

Kinaesthetics

You learn to play a musical instrument by using your sense of touch. Your fingers remember the correct positions and pressures. Also, you can reinforce other memories by adding some sort of motion to them. For example, some people beat out time while memorizing. You might not want everyone to see you do this (they might just get the wrong idea about your sanity), but it does work.

Learning it parrot fashion

Repeat after me: 0795634. Say it again, and again, and again. If you work at it for a couple of minutes, you'll find that the memory sticks – but not for long. It's doubtful whether, without using some other method, you would be able to remember those numbers this time tomorrow. But that's OK because there are some things we just don't want to remember for very long. So, if you look up a phone number and want to remember it just long enough to get to the phone and punch the buttons, repetition is a good technique. If, however, you've just met someone you think might

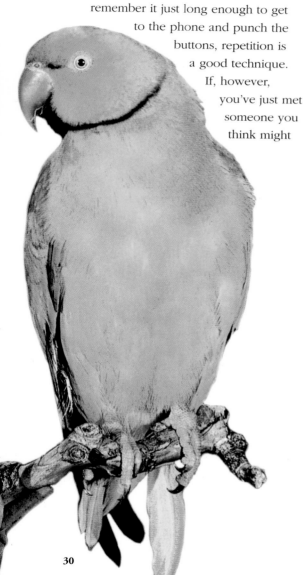

PLAY IT AGAIN, SAM
Memories that you want to keep fresh should be reviewed regularly. After you have used the techniques in this book for a while, you'll build up a library of memories and, from time to time, you need to test yourself again. You can do this in any scrap of spare time you have, for example while travelling to work, or even while doing some other task such as mowing the lawn or cooking dinner. This reviewing procedure needn't be boring and can actually be quite a good way to relax and forget the stresses of the day.

become the love of your life and have been given his or her phone number, this is not a safe way to commit it to memory.

When my kids were really young, they would prepare for spelling tests by repeating the spellings until they got them all right. In those days, I knew less about memory than I do now, so, because I'd been taught to learn my spellings parrot fashion as well, I went along with it. The result? They both got excellent marks in their spelling tests, BUT by the next week they had forgotten everything they'd supposedly learnt.

Repetition forms part of all the other techniques you will learn and, used in combination with those techniques, it is very powerful; on its own it is only a temporary fix.

As an experiment, we'll see just how many digits you can commit to memory using ONLY the repetition method. Here's a series of 50 digits in groups of five.

There is another important use for repetition, however, and that is in getting other people to remember something. I used to study Spanish at a local community college. People came from surrounding villages; one of which was called Over. Every time anyone mentioned that they came from Over, the teacher would say 'sobre' (the Spanish for 'over'). He said it every lesson and, by the end of the year, if there was one word of Spanish that everyone remembered permanently it was 'sobre'. The limitation of this technique is that you can only get people to remember things they want to remember. If you repeat something they don't want to remember, it'll just bounce off like water off a duck's back. For example, I frequently tell my kids to tidy up and turn off TVs, hair straighteners, CD players, lights and so on before they go to school. Several thousand repetitions have so far failed to do the trick.

3	5	9	2	0
4	1	0	6	8
5	1	1	9	3
8	7	3	0	1
3	4	2	0	4
5	2	8	6	9
2	0	3	7	8
1	5	5	0	3
6	3	7	9	2
5	3	8	3	8

Remember, the rule is that you must only use repetition to memorize these numbers. See how many you can remember and how long you can retain your sequence. You'll probably be disappointed, but don't worry – this is only a minor way of memorizing.

A memory is what is left when something happens and does not completely unhappen.
Edward de Bono

God gave us memories that we might have roses in December.
J. M. Barrie, *Courage*

There's always something there to remind me

When you were young, you may have had quirky tricks, such as tying a knot in the corner of your handkerchief to help you remember simple tasks or chores. Physical reminders like this are a quick and easy way to get you to remember something simple that might otherwise slip your mind. The hanky knot is invaluable for reminding you to take your kids to the dentist. Some people use methods such as a rubber band wound around one finger (rather uncomfortable and too obvious) or a sticking plaster covering a non-existent cut.

Physical reminders can be extended from your person to your surroundings. Leaving some familiar object out of its normal place can act as a memory trigger. For most of us, this technique can work at a simple level (car keys left on the coffee table (instead of on the key rack) can tell you to take the car for servicing), but if you leave too many reminders around they might become confusing. Some families get so used to communicating in this way, that they leave quite complicated 'notes' for each other that no one else could ever understand. For example, someone might leave a stone misplaced near the front door to tell other family members that a spare set of house keys has been hidden in the potting shed. Cunning, eh?

This is Jim's house. The book lying open on his desk is to remind him to go the library. The car keys have been left on top of the computer to remind him to get the car serviced, and the picture of his wife is upside down, not because he's careless, but because tomorrow is her birthday and he must remember to buy her a present.

ATTACK ON ALL FRONTS AT ONCE
Don't use just one technique to remember something – try to use several. Looking, listening and doing methods should all be combined for the best result. For an example of how to do this, go to 'Learn the kings and queens of England' on pages 92–93 and look at the hints there.

Memory is a child walking along a seashore. You never can tell what small pebble it will pick up and store away among its treasured things.
Pierce Harris, *Atlanta Journal*

We do not remember days; we remember moments.
Cesare Pavese, *The Burning Brand*

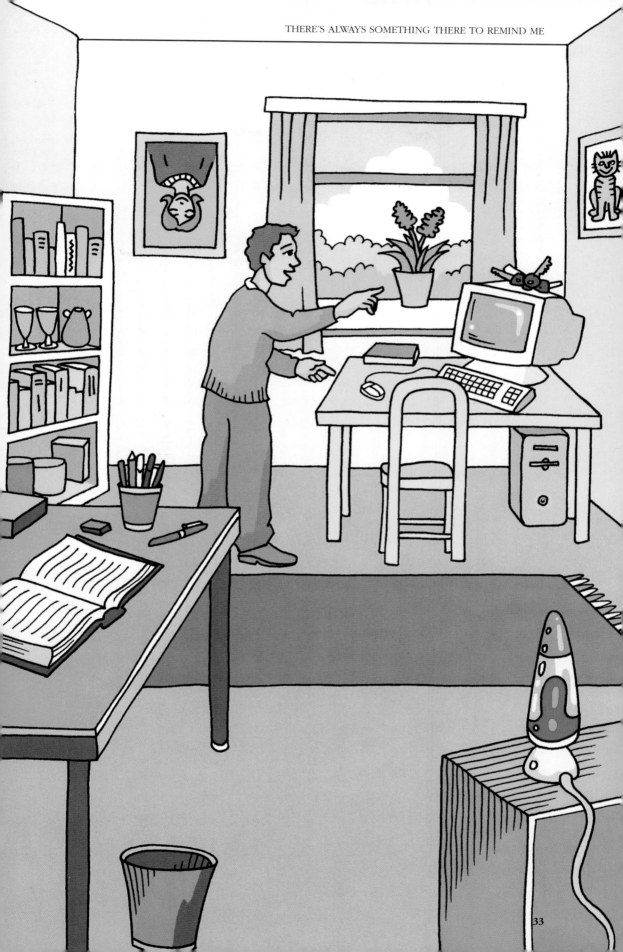

It's all in the mind

Can you visualize your house? Yes, almost certainly you can. You probably know every nook and cranny of it and could find your way around blindfold. This is what makes it an excellent device for memorizing.

Let's say you are going shopping. One way of remembering the things you need to buy would be to imagine the objects around the house. For example, a newspaper lying on your virtual kitchen table will remind you to go and buy *The Times*. You can strengthen the memory bond by making the objects appropriate to the places they are left – a bag of sugar near a photo of your little daughter (isn't she sweet?) and a bag of lemons next to the photo of your mother-in-law ...

Give it a try. Take the following list and place the items in your virtual house (or another place you feel comfortable with):

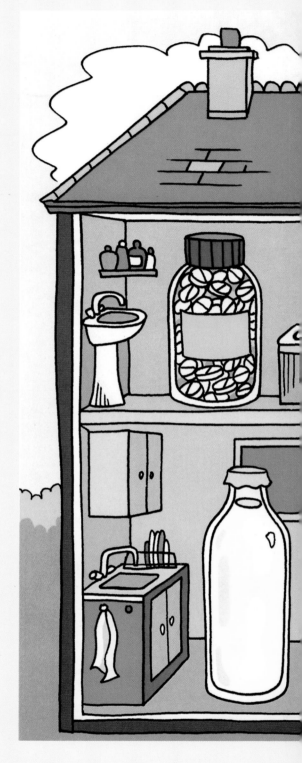

Newspaper	**Fertilizer**
Painkillers	**Guitar strings**
Chocolate bar	**Oranges**
Milk	**TV listings**
Sugar	**magazine**
Cookies	**Barbecue charcoal**
Apples	**Cut flowers**
Potatoes	**Knitting wool**
Breakfast cereal	**Sausages**
Sticking plasters	**Toothpaste**
Weedkiller	

Check through your list several times until you're sure you can remember every item clearly. Always walk around your virtual house in the same order. This adds a very important element of ritual to your memorizing.

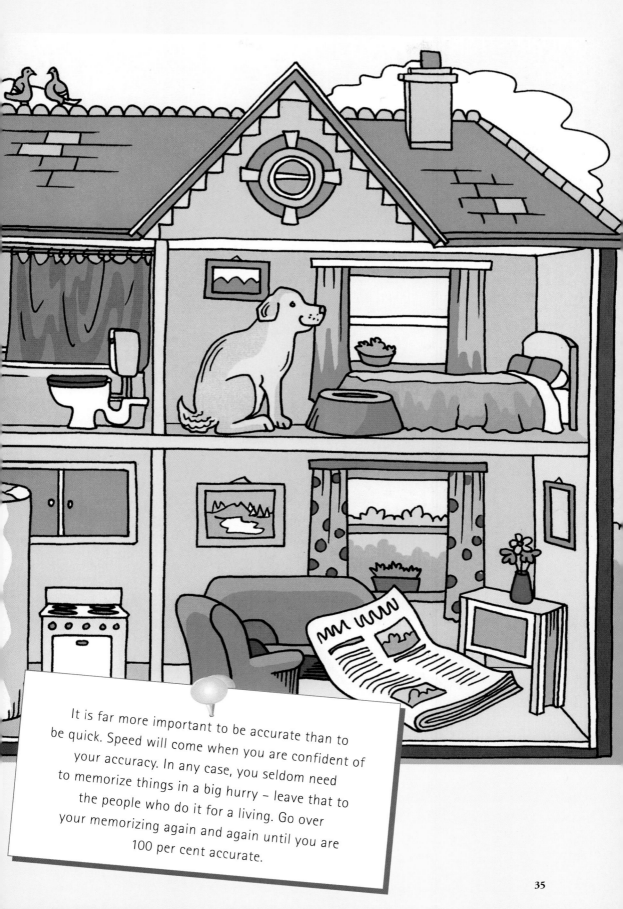

It is far more important to be accurate than to be quick. Speed will come when you are confident of your accuracy. In any case, you seldom need to memorize things in a big hurry – leave that to the people who do it for a living. Go over your memorizing again and again until you are 100 per cent accurate.

I want to tell you a story

One way of remembering things is to combine them into a silly story. Note the word 'silly'. The sillier the story, the more likely you are to remember it. For example, using the items pictured, you could come up with something like this.

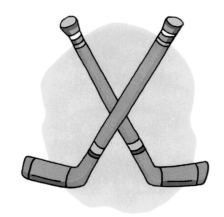

I was waking on stilts (that looked like **hockey sticks**)

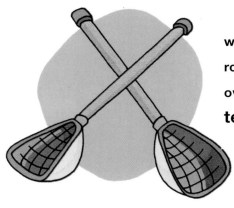

when I **lacrossed** the road and tripped over a heap of **tennis balls**.

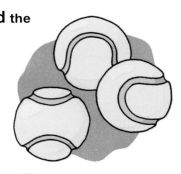

My intentions were **foiled** because I crashed into a **fence**,

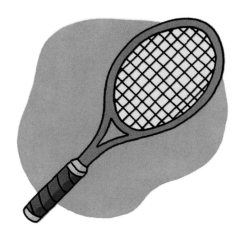

which made an enormous **racket**.

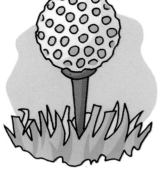

After that I needed some **tea**,

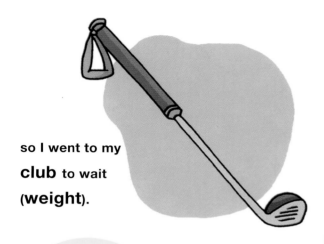

so I went to my **club** to wait **(weight)**.

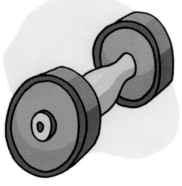

KEEP IT WACKY
You don't remember sensible things because they're just too boring. You do remember wacky things. Use wild associations, crazy rhymes, and weird visual images. My father taught me the alphabet by getting me to sing it to the tune of the Ode to Joy from Beethoven's Ninth Symphony. You think that's a crazy thing to teach a little kid? I loved it! Try singing it in the shower and you'll see what I mean.

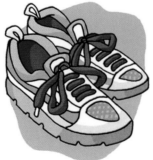

No one offered me a lift so I **ran** home,

Stupid? Undoubtedly. But *memorable*. Try it out for yourself. Come up with your own story and I bet that within a few minutes you'll be able to remember the whole list without omitting a single item.

The only problem with this method is that it does confine you to remembering all the items in the same order. If someone asked you, 'Does the tennis racket come before or after the golf clubs?', you'd probably have to run through the whole story to make sure.

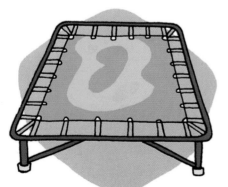

which left me feeling full of **bounce**.

Memory is a complicated thing, a relative to truth, but not its twin.
Barbara Kingsolver, *Animal Dreams*

Rhythm and rhyme

When no one's listening, try singing the nursery rhyme 'Jack and Jill Went Up the Hill'. Go on! Just for me. One thing I'll guarantee, you haven't forgotten the words or the tune. That's because rhythm and rhyme are very, very, very strong memory glue. If you want to remember something forever, set it to music with a good, strong rhythm. In olden times, the bards would not just tell old stories, they would sing them. That's how they remembered all those interminable tales of heroes, gods and beautiful maidens. If I ask you to tell me a well-known story like, say, Peter Pan, you'll probably be able to give me a précis; but the whole thing, word for word? I doubt it. But you can learn huge chunks of Shakespeare by heart because that's poetry and the rhythm helps you, even though much of the language is unfamiliar.

Some people complain about being made to learn poetry by heart at school, but I loved it. Have a go at Walter Scott's 'Lochinvar'. What, all of it? Yes, why not? You'll find that because it is real old-fashioned poetry with strong rhythm and rhyme, you'll memorize it easily and, more to the point, permanently.

Instructions

☆ There is no magic trick to learning things that come with rhythm and rhyme built in. The fact is that our minds naturally store anything that comes in this form. That's why kids can learn endless pop songs and be word perfect in all of them.

☆ All you have to do is split the thing into chunks (the Scott poem works in couplets, so that's the best way to learn it).

☆ Just keep going over it until the rhythm and rhyme embed themselves in your memory.

The past is never dead, it is not even past.
William Faulkner

A happy childhood can't be cured. Mine'll hang around my neck like a rainbow, that's all, instead of a noose.
Hortense Calisher, *Queenie*, 1971

Lochinvar by Sir Walter Scott

O young Lochinvar is come out of the west,
Through all the wide Border his steed was the best;
And save his good broadsword he weapons had none,
He rode all unarm'd, and he rode all alone,
So faithful in love, and so dauntless in War,
There never was knight like the young Lochinvar.

He staid not for brake, and he stopp'd not for stone,
He swam the Eske river where ford there was none;
But ere he alighted at Netherby gate,
The bride had consented, the gallant came late:
For a laggard in love, and a dastard in war,
Was to wed the fair Ellen of brave Lochinvar.

So boldly he enter'd the Netherby Hall,
Among bride's-men, and kinsmen, and brothers and all:
Then spoke the bride's father, his hand on his sword,
(For the poor craven bridegroom said never a word),
"O come ye in peace here, or come ye in war,
Or to dance at our bridal, young Lord Lochinvar?"

"I long woo'd your daughter, my suit you denied;
Love swells like the Solway, but ebbs like its tide
And now I am come, with this lost love of mine,
To lead but one measure, drink one cup of wine,
There are maidens in Scotland more lovely by far,
That would gladly be bride to the young Lochinvar."

The bride kiss'd the goblet: the knight took it up,
He quaff'd off the wine, and he threw down the cup.
She look'd down to blush, and she look'd up to sigh.
With a smile on her lips and a tear in her eye,
He took her soft hand, ere her mother could bar,
"Now tread we a measure!" said young Lochinvar.

So stately his form, and so lovely her face,
That never a hall such a gailiard did grace;
While her mother did fret, and her father did fume
And the bridegroom stood dangling his bonnet and plume;
And the bride-maidens whisper'd, "'twere better by far
To have match'd our fair cousin with young Lochinvar."

One touch to her hand, and one word in her ear,
When they reach'd the hall-door, and the charger stood near;
So light to the croupe the fair lady he swung,
So light to the saddle before her he sprung!
"She is won! We are gone, over bank, bush, and scaur;
They'll have fleet steeds that follow," quoth young Lochinvar.

There was mounting 'mong Graemes of the Netherby clan;
Forsters, Fenwicks, and Musgraves, they rode and they ran:
There was racing and chasing on Cannobie Lee,
But the lost bride of Netherby ne'er did they see.
So daring in love, and so dauntless in war,
Have ye e'er heard of gallant like young Lochinvar?

GIVE ME A BREAK!

It is important to take breaks during a memorization task. The mind works in mysterious ways, and one of them is that it keeps on working even when you think it has stopped. If you start a task today, and then stop and get a night's sleep, you'll find that during the night your mind has been mulling over the memory and by the next day. Your performance will have improved. If you don't take breaks, you'll get tired and stale and your task will be longer and more arduous.

I can see it all!

Some people are born visualizers. Their imagination is full of vivid pictures and vibrant colours. My visual memory, on the other hand, looks like a collection of rather faded picture postcards. If you have a really good visual memory, you can make use of it in a number of ways. One of them is to play Memory Lane.

Think of the street where you live (or any other street that you know really well). In your mind's eye, walk down the street depositing items that you want to remember in all the front gardens. You can include just about anything. In our illustration the man is reminding himself to take an umbrella when he goes to work (rain is forecast), get in a round of golf when he comes home, and buy butter, sugar and tea. There's a list of 'Things To Do' outside the local shop. Finally, he reminds himself to go to a friend's party where he will book tickets for Hawaii (his

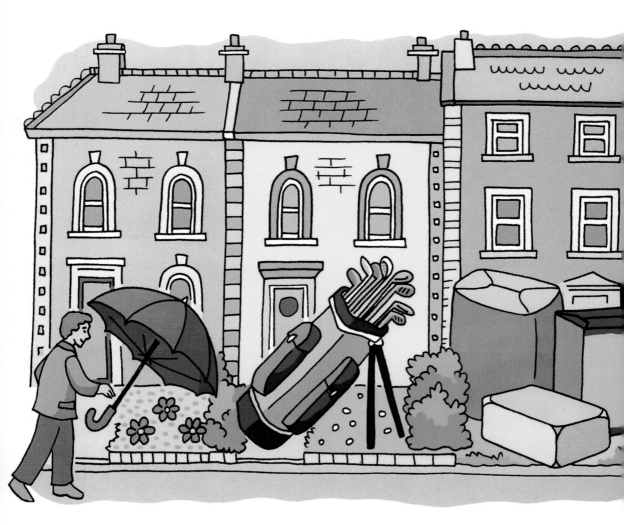

friend is in the travel business and gets him a discount).

You can extend this technique as much as you like. Some people, for example, learn dates by mentally carving them on a stone timeline. Another use for visual memory is in remembering faces and places. If visual memories work for you (there's no particular trick to doing it), you just have to remember to do it! If you're visiting a new town for the first time, make sure you keep a visual record of the route you take through the town so that you can find your way back to where you parked the car.

Divide and conquer

Never attempt to memorize large chunks of material in one go. Split large tasks into smaller elements. If there is a natural split (the stanzas of a poem, for example) it is helpful, but if not, just create an artificial division to suit yourself. To see this technique in action, look at 'Presidents of the USA' on pages 98–101.

In memory's telephoto lens, far objects are magnified.
John Updike

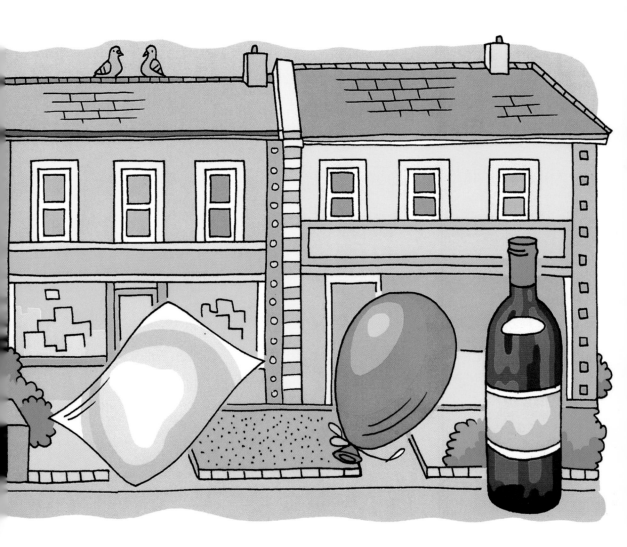

Learning by doing

For some people, the very best way to learn about something is to go and do it. They get more information from that than they would from any amount of book learning. This ability lends itself to a whole area of memory techniques based on doing, which are sometimes called 'kinaesthetic techniques'.

When I was young, I went to a school that had strong views about pupils bringing the right books and equipment with them for lessons. The words, 'Sorry, I forgot', were not met with a smile. So, how did I manage to avoid trouble? I constructed a ritual for filling my school bag every evening. It was very complicated, but that was precisely the reason it worked. Not only did each book and item of equipment have its own place, but each one had to be put in the bag in the correct order. It soon became a virtual impossibility to forget anything, because if I did, the ritual didn't feel right and I'd soon spot my oversight.

That is one sort of ritual, but there are other much more complicated and useful ones.

The past is malleable and flexible, changing as our recollection interprets and re-explains what has happened.

Peter Berger

There are lots of people who mistake their imagination for their memory.

Josh Billings

When something that we do regularly is considered important, one way of making sure it all goes to plan is to turn it into ritual. Churches have been good at this for centuries. So have other institutions such as monarchies. A nice bit of ritual binds the community together and reminds everyone of their place in the grand scheme. But how is this relevant to your quest for a better memory?

The army is often derided for teaching people to do things by numbers. But this is actually a very good and practical use of ritual. How else would you teach a youngster who has little formal education (and may not be too bright) to strip down a complicated device such as a machine gun, correct a jammed mechanism, and put it all back together again, without losing any of the pieces? Ritual, that's

ORDER, ORDER!
When you learn a list of things (telephone numbers, for example) make sure that you frequently change the order in which you rehearse them. If you don't, there is a strong risk that you will be committing the order itself to memory. If that happens, you will find that you have to go through the whole list every time you want to find one item. So, when you rehearse your list, mix it up so that the order never forms part of your memory pattern.

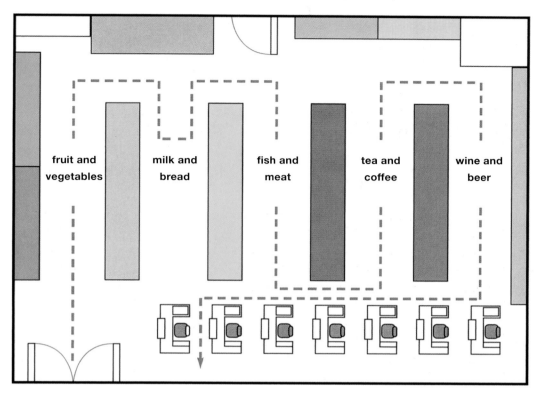

Supermarket routines

how. Once they learn to do it by numbers, they will never forget, even when under fire and in a highly stressed state. It has become impossible to leave out one of the numbered stages.

My wife has another sort of ritual. When she visits the supermarket she always makes exactly the same tour. Most of us buy more or less the same stuff each week, but with some changes (for example, you probably don't need razors every week). But once you've committed the order to memory, you no longer have to think about it and can concentrate your energy on remembering any changes to the usual routine (for example, maybe this week you fancy wine instead of beer). You can extend your ritual to cover not just the supermarket, but all the other places you normally have to visit. The ritual makes it very unlikely you'll forget anything important. Some people might object that shopping this way is rather boring and mechanical. To counter that, we save the fun stuff (new clothes, CDs, etc.) until last so that we can enjoy them at our leisure.

Don't knock ritual! It is an effortless way to remember complicated information without mistakes. Think, for example, of how you drive a manual car. Do you consciously think: apply brakes, slow down, change gear, check mirror, look both ways at junction? No, of course you don't. Once you can drive, the whole process becomes automatic. No matter what the circumstances on the road, the appropriate ritual will cut in. The only time you'll be flummoxed is if you get into a violent skid and haven't bothered to learn the technique for dealing with a skid safely.

The gentle touch

Do you remember showing some new possession (a camera, for example) to a friend for the first time? He says, 'Oh, let's have a look!' and takes it from you, apparently to look closer. But as well as looking, he is also feeling. For some reason, we are a bit coy about our habit of learning through touch. We actually would like to touch all sorts of things (especially other people) just to get to know them better, to quite literally get a feel for them. The sense of touch is delicate but also very powerful.

Touch does not just inform us of things that are going on right now, but it also involves a specialized kind of memory. A blind friend once showed me how he could run his fingers over the cards in a pack and identify many of them just by the way they felt: odd irregularities, creases and bent corners, which would be just about invisible to a sighted person, were picked out unerringly by his heightened sense of touch.

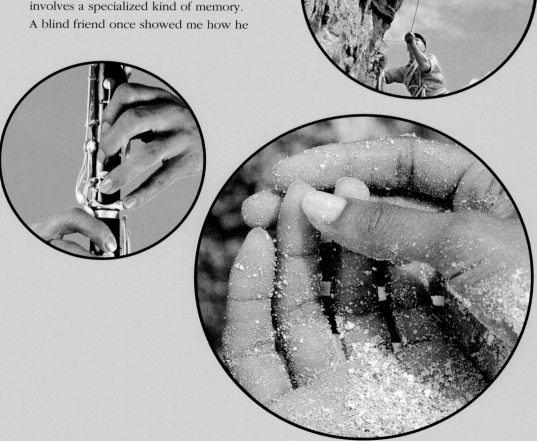

Although our sense of touch is innate, like all other senses it can be improved by practice. You need to spend some time quite deliberately feeling objects and trying to identify them just from touch. Some work depends entirely on a well-

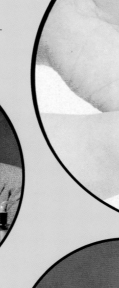

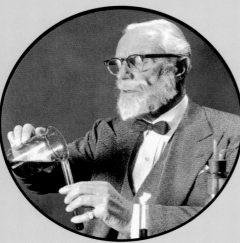

developed touch memory. For example, a bomb disposal officer is trained to do this sort of work largely by the memory of how things feel. It is not always possible to open up a bomb and take a good look inside, so he needs to be able to feel his way around. A touch in the wrong place could put a very sudden end to his career.

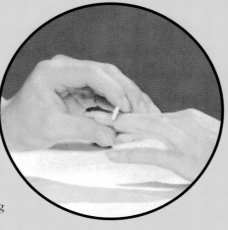

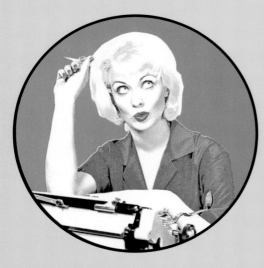

It's surprising how much memory is built around things unnoticed at the time.
Barbara Kingsolver, *Animal Dreams*

To look backward for a while is to refresh the eye, to restore it, and to render it the more fit for its prime function of looking forward.
Margaret Fairless Barber,
The Roadmender

Eidetic memory

What used to be called photographic memory is now known by the term 'eidetic memory'. Some people can look briefly at an object, design or document and then reproduce it in minute detail, just as though their mind had taken a photograph of it. As you would imagine, there is huge controversy surrounding this whole topic. Some psychologists are strong believers in eidetic memory, whilst others have doubts, or even deny that there is any such phenomenon.

It seems beyond question that certain individuals do have a greater-than-average ability to remember things they have seen. One of my aunts, who was trained as a dressmaker, had the useful ability to copy any dress after looking at it for only a very short time, She built up a thriving business turning out imitations of dresses she had seen pictured at society weddings, or worn by film stars. A flick through the pages of the gossip magazines or, better still, a few minutes spent in the presence

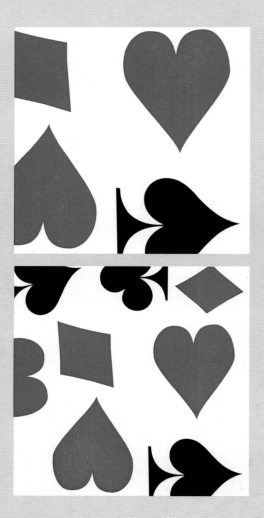

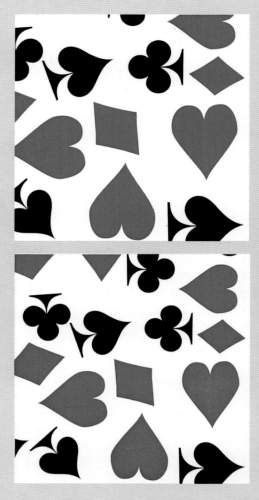

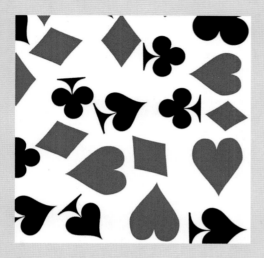
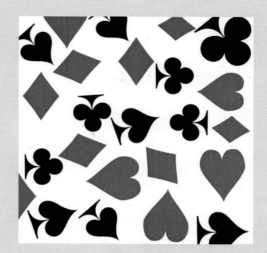

of the actual dress, and she could make you a perfect copy

The point is, could you learn to do this; or do you have to be born with the ability? Let's see! The drawings on these pages start out as quite simple, but get increasingly complex. Look at each drawing (for as long as you need). Then put the book aside and try to reproduce the drawing in as much detail as possible.

TRAIN YOUR EIDETIC MEMORY
There are numerous free computer games, available on the Internet to help train your eidetic memory. Simply search under the words 'eidetic memory training' and you will find a wide choice of programs on offer.

One of the most moving aspects of life is how long the deepest memories stay with us. It is as if the individual memory is enclosed in a greater, which even in the night of our forgetfulness stands like an angel with folded wings ready, at the moment of acknowledged need, to guide us back to the lost spoor of meaning.
Laurens Van Der Post

Our memories are card indexes consulted, and then put back in disorder by authorities who we do not control.
Cyril Connolly, *The Unquiet Grave*

Mozart memories?

Much has been written about the so-called 'Mozart effect' and the whole area has been infected by controversy and commercialism. I don't want to argue about whether little kids can have their IQs boosted by listening to Mozart, simply because it is not relevant to our purpose. What I do want to discuss is whether any sort of music can aid concentration and memory.

Many people like to use music as a background to any sort of work. Runners in the park, kids doing homework, workers on assembly lines and shoppers in supermarkets all receive a daily dose of background music. I regularly visit the design studio of one of my publishers and see the designers hunched over their Macs, each in his or her own private world of music. But does the music help or distract?

What follows are my personal views and I make no claims other than they are based on my own experiences, and those of my family and students I have worked with in my creative writing classes. If you disagree, feel free to do so and listen to whatever you please. If it works for you, it works.

The only thing I would absolutely advise against, when trying to memorize, is having a TV on anywhere near you. If you can see it, you will not be able to concentrate on the work in hand. Even the most witless game show or soap looks entrancing when the alternative is to do some work. If you can only hear the Tv, it's not much better – you'll be wondering, even if only at the back of your mind, what is happening on screen. You'll almost certainly give in at some point and go to take a quick peek. You may return to your work (or not), but in any case your concentration will be broken.

Music is far more a matter of personal taste. My kids swear that they can revise to the strains of heavy rock. I'm sure that you can do some tasks to music but I doubt that you can marshal all your concentration when you are listening to something loud and lively. Having said that, I must confess that I'm writing this to the strains of Pink Floyd, and my concentration is unbroken so far.

So how about classical music? Like many people, I enjoy popular classics. I can happily listen to *The Four Seasons* or *Scheherazade*, but it's not the sort of music I'd choose to work to – until recently, that is. I read an article about the way in which classical music (any classical music) could increase your concentration and improve memory. Since it was strictly relevant to this book I gave it a try and, to my surprise, it worked very well indeed. I recommend it to you. You don't even have to like the music. But it does create a calm atmosphere where you will find concentration easier and where memories will stick. And the quicker you learn, the sooner you can get back to the TV.

> Don't just memorize at odd moments. Plan a session, decide how long it will last and what you will achieve. Decide when you will take a rest.

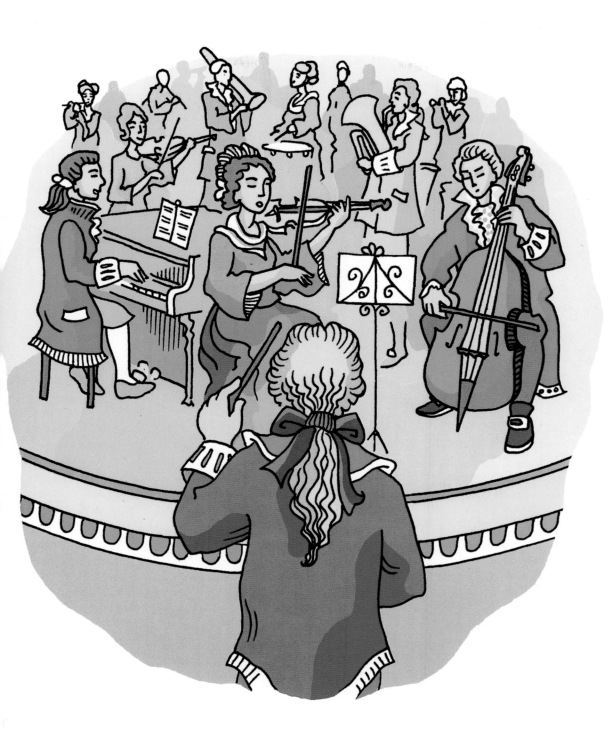

***Every day your memory grows dimmer/
it doesn't haunt me like it did before.***

Bob Dylan

You are not a computer

Some people maintain that the brain works like some sort of super-computer. They even talk about removing faulty programs and replacing them with new, improved ones. Piffle! The brain is not at all like a computer. Don't be fooled into believing this sort of nonsense. Your memory works in a mysterious and highly complex fashion. It needs careful training and maintenance. You do NOT have

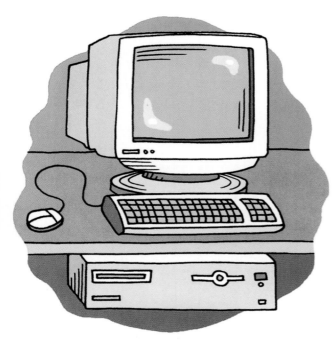

It is singular how soon we lose the impression of what ceases to be constantly before us. A year impairs, a lustre obliterates. There is little distinct left without an effort of memory, then indeed the lights are rekindled for a moment – but who can be sure that the Imagination is not the torch-bearer?

Lord Byron

Computer

☆ No sense of humour

☆ 100 per cent recall on hard disk, floppies and CD-ROM

☆ Can share memories with other computers

☆ No visual memory (but can recognize photos when encoded)

☆ No emotional reaction to memory

☆ No creativity

☆ Will only recall what the human operator asks for

☆ Unable to memorize smells

☆ Memories are in no particular order of importance

☆ Very limited ability to learn from experience

☆ Does not learn by touch – Requires no rest

☆ Requires no food (but needs electricity in order to function)

☆ Has no emotions

☆ Will recall any memory upon request

☆ All memories remain just as they were when recorded

a hard disk in your head. Here are the main differences between the way you memorize and the way a computer does it.

Human

☆ Sense of humour (in most models)

☆ Fallible and capable of forgetting even important data

☆ Able to share memories with other humans

☆ Strong visual memory

☆ Memory used to spark off creative tasks

☆ Quirky memory that recalls data not asked for

☆ Memorizes smells

☆ Memories are roughly ranked according to importance

☆ Learns greatly from experience

☆ Can learn complicated tasks by touch alone

☆ Must sleep or die

☆ Has complicated dietary requirements that can affect memory

☆ Memories are strongly linked to emotions

☆ May resist recalling painful memories

☆ Can add sentimental gloss to memories (the 'Good Old Days' effect)

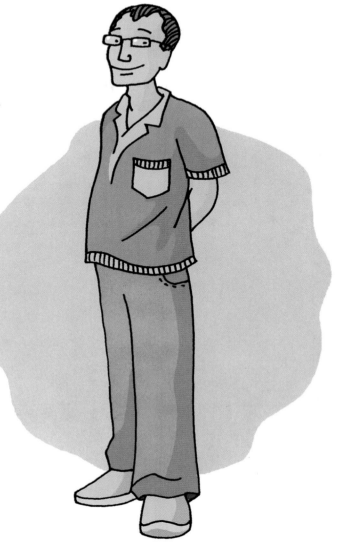

TESTING, TESTING, TESTING
It is very easy to convince yourself that you remember something when you are really not yet word-perfect. To get over this difficulty, you should get someone to test you whenever possible.

Inability to remember

If you find yourself unable to retain information, there may be several possible reasons. The main one is usually stress. You will never be able to memorize if you let yourself get stressed. Memory is like sex – you have to be in the right mood, and that means feeling happy, relaxed and enthusiastic about what you are doing.

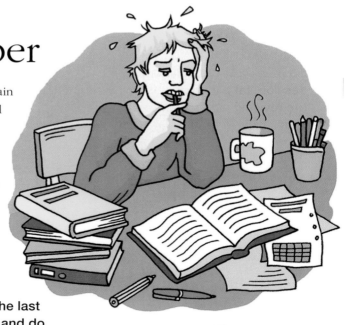

☆ Do NOT leave revising to the last minute. Start in good time and do a little – thoroughly – each day. It is far better to learn a little bit well than to try to cram in a whole lot and make a mess of it. To get it all done on time, you must plan your revision well.

☆ Do things to ensure you're in a good mood. Have some snacks and drinks (non-alcoholic) nearby to reward yourself for your efforts. If you like music, put some on at a low volume (you won't revise properly if you have to contend with loud music).

☆ Make sure that you are not too warm or too cold.

☆ Allow plenty of fresh air into the room. A stuffy room makes you drowsy and messes up your ability to concentrate.

☆ Keep other members of the family away and get someone to answer the phone and take messages for you.

TRYING TO FORGET

One of the ways in which you differ from a computer is that your memories cannot be deleted at will. Memories that are not reviewed regularly will fade eventually. Memories that are of no further interest (like a once-only telephone number) will vanish without trace. Unpleasant memories have a habit of sticking just because they are unpleasant. The harder you struggle against such memories, the harder they are to erase. My uncle was with troops who liberated a Nazi death camp, and he struggled with the memory for the next forty years.

The only way (and it's by no means infallible) to deal with such memories is to review them when they resurface.

☆ **To revise successfully, you need to concentrate for at least half an hour to an hour. Too little will do you no good and too much will make you stale. After each session, take a break. When you are revising hard for an exam, you can get in three or four one-hour sessions a day, then go out and do something completely different.**

If you really can't remember, despite your best efforts, you need to ask yourself why. Are you studying something you really hate just to please your parents? Are you in a career that no longer interests you? Are you afraid of failing your exams? If there is some unresolved issue that is stopping you from memorizing successfully, then unless you face and resolve it, you will find your efforts constantly frustrated.

What's stopping you?

A major cause of faulty memory is lack of understanding. Certain things can be learnt parrot fashion, whether you understand them or not (though almost any attempt at memorization is improved by understanding). For example, you can learn the dates of all the battles in the American Civil War by rote if you want to. But how much better it would be if you understood the background, who was fighting and why. When you have that sort of framework to hang the information on, it is far easier to make it stick.

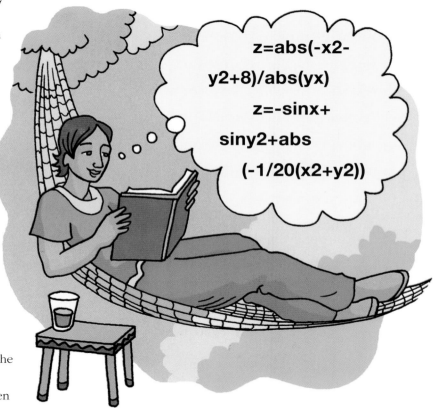

Some things just cannot be learnt without understanding them. Science without understanding becomes a jumble of weird symbols and figures. Literature becomes soulless and without meaning. If you master the background to a subject, the information will be easier to assimilate.

Everybody needs his memories. They keep the wolf of insignificance from the door.
Saul Bellow

Ah, yes! I remember that smell!

Smell is the strongest memory key of all. This is strange when you consider that, compared to other animals, our sense of smell is quite frail. Nevertheless, we have all had the experience of a sudden aroma taking us back to some place we loved or hated years before. Chalk dust can evoke school classrooms, the smell of chlorine conjures up swimming lessons long past, and strawberries have a smell inseparable from hot summer days.

The smell trigger is highly personal. Although most readers will relate to at least some of the smells given off by the items below (because they are very common ones), we all have our own special triggers. I react strongly to the smell of the herb coriander (cilantro). It reminds me of my time teaching in Thailand, when it was served with virtually every meal. It has a powerful smell which, until I was used to it, I found rather

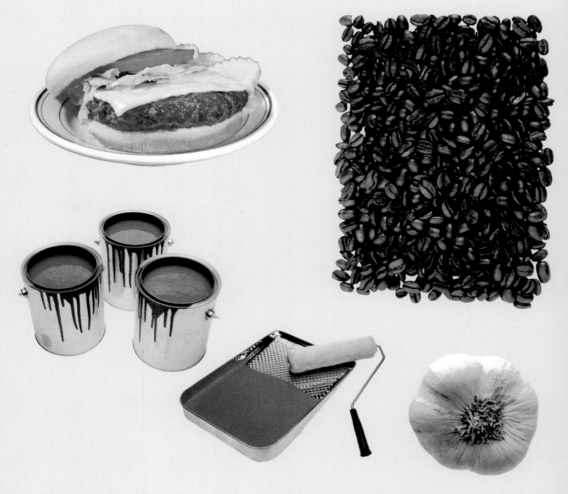

offensive. Then I got to like it, and now the smell reminds me of delicious Thai meals I've enjoyed in the past.

It is frustrating that the smell trigger cannot be used to help us store information. It doesn't provoke the right kind of memory. Smell is closely linked to emotion rather than the recall of facts. It might help you to remember places, people, or things that made you happy, sad, angry, lovelorn, or amused; sadly, it cannot remind you of, say, the names of the Presidents of the USA.

Is there any practical use for the smell trigger? It is useful for creating moods (as anyone who owns an oil burner, or who regularly uses incense, will testify).

You could use it as an adjunct to other memorization methods by introducing aromas that you find agreeable and which put you in a relaxed mood.

CONFIDENCE

Probably when someone gives you an address, phone number or any other important information, you rush at once to write it down. Don't! Learn to have confidence in your memory. The more practice you have at remembering, the more you remember. Have confidence in your ability and you'll soon find that it is justified.

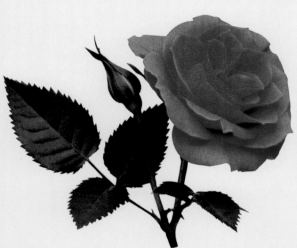

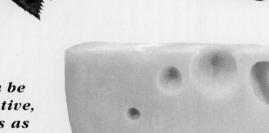

The sense of smell can be extraordinarily evocative, bringing back pictures as sharp as photographs, of scenes that had left the conscious mind.

Thalassa Cruso,
To Everything There is a Season

Ah, yes! I remember it well!

You might remember a number from the musical *Gigi* in which an old man and his sometime lady-friend recall their first date. He gets all the details wrong and she corrects him but, even so, he always replies, 'Ah, yes! I remember it well!' And he does! This is an excellent example of what is now called False Memory Syndrome. I'll give you another. When I was a boy in Scotland, we used to go to Craiglockhart golf course in Edinburgh for tobogganing. It was five minutes' walk from my house. I remember the scene vividly. The clubhouse was on the right and the golf course swept away majestically to the left. It was a really excellent place to ride a toboggan. Recently, I went back after forty something years and found the scene exactly as I remembered it. Except for this: the clubhouse was actually on the left and the golf course swept away to the right! It was not that I'd come in from another direction, because I'd found my old house and followed the exact route I'd taken so often as a kid. But there we are – a false memory.

We don't know a lot about how false memories happen, but research suggests that they can be encouraged very easily. In a recent experiment, volunteers listened to a description of experiences they could not possibly have had (though they were unaware of this). For example, a group of British volunteers were told of an incident in which a skin test was carried out by scraping a sample of skin from the little finger. (This particular technique is simply not used in the UK, though it is common in the US, so there was

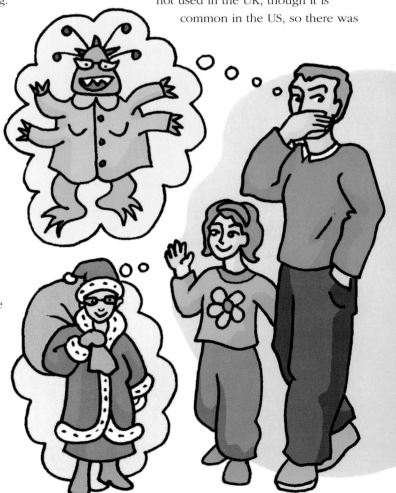

no way any of these people could have had it done to them.) Some members of the group subsequently went on to form very clear memories of having had such a test taken.

False Memory Syndrome can be simply odd and even quite amusing, but it does have a sinister side. Some psychotherapists have made a fortune helping clients to recover memories of sexual abuse during childhood. Theoretically, these were memories that had been buried deep in the psyche because of the trauma associated with them. Increasingly, however, it seems that a proportion of such patients have simply been encouraged to form false memories of events that never took place.

If you want to see False Memory Syndrome in action for yourself, try this experiment. Ask your family or a group of friends to write a description of an event you shared. It could be a party, a family gathering, or an outing of some sort. Not only will the individuals all remember the event slightly differently, but the chances are that at least one person will come up with a scene that the others are all quite sure never took place.

Nostalgia is like a grammar lesson: you find the present tense and the past perfect.
Anon

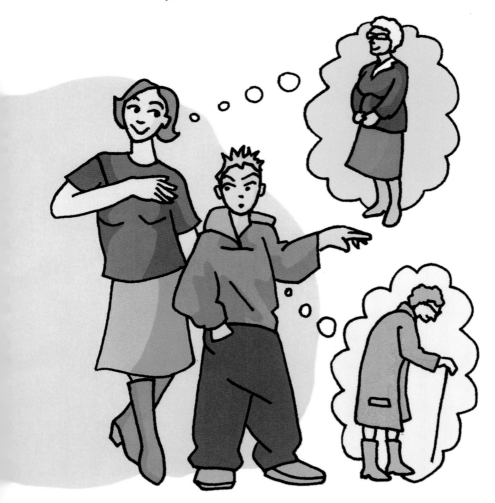

The long and winding road

This is an exercise in using your long-term memory. There is nothing you need to do to form this type of memory – it happens automatically. Your unconscious will simply file stuff away without any reference to your conscious desires at all. This can be quite inconvenient. Sometimes you may find yourself desperate to remember an incident from long ago, only to find that you can't dredge it up. At other times, you'll find yourself plagued with memories that are either quite useless and distracting or, even worse, decidedly unpleasant.

What to do? It is a good idea, every now and again, to deliberately stimulate long-term memory. There are several ways of doing this and you should use all of them. One is simply to sit and recollect incidents from your past. You can just ramble aimlessly down memory lane if you want to, or you can pick out a specific train of thought (school days, jobs you have held, old friends, former lovers, whatever takes your fancy). Just let your mind meander where it will. The more relaxed you feel, the more likely you are to have a good experience. An extra way of stimulating the flow of memory is to either write your thoughts down (you don't have to be an expert writer, notes will do just

as well), or to recount your experiences to a relative or friend. If you do use someone as a recipient for memories, make sure it is a person who is both willing and trustworthy.

Another way to get the long-term memory centre working is to look through mementoes and photographs, or to visit places that you used to frequent long ago. This is obviously a very powerful stimulant and you'll probably find that once you do it, the flow of memory will turn into a flood.

Finally, you might try talking to friends, relatives, colleagues and acquaintances from your past. People are often very keen to do this (as can be seen from the success of various websites that encourage people to get back in contact with their former friends).

For most people, there are considerable benefits in keeping their long term

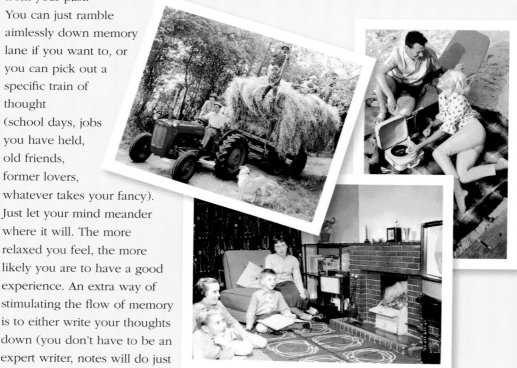

memory in good repair. It aids mental health by reinforcing our sense of identity,

reassuring us about who we are and how we fit into our own personal life story: It can provide a feeling of warmth and security that is far better than anything you can get from pills.

Just one word of warning – if your life is full of unresolved conflicts, unhappy memories and repressed traumas, you should only carry out this exercise in the company of a trained professional.

To help you begin your journey, try the suggestions below. They will give you some preliminary thoughts that will launch your voyage of exploration in the right direction. We tried a questionnaire a bit like this earlier in the book, but this one is more ambitious and, as you are doing it entirely for your own private interest, you should take your time over it and not let yourself feel rushed.

Considering these questions will almost certainly put you in a mood where other memories come flooding out. This mood of reverie may persist for hours or even days.

1 Write down or talk about your very favourite memory. With luck, you will have lots of good ones to choose from, and deciding which is the best will be part of the fun. Examining memories will also set off trains of thought that you will find interesting and rewarding.

2 Discuss, with yourself or others, who is the one person in your life you would like to meet again. Why is that person so important to you? Recall as many events associated with that person as you can. Once you start, you will find other memories begin to push forward into your consciousness.

3 List your greatest achievements. These need not be grand – you don't have to have climbed Everest or explored the Amazon rainforest. Little things will do as long as they mean a lot to you.

4 Name a favourite TV programme from when you were a child. Remember as many details as you can. Just what was it you enjoyed so much? Would you still enjoy it now if you were able to see are-run?

5 Write something about pets you had in the past. Pet memories are often sweet and sad at the same time. They are also a very potent reminder of times past.

6 Discuss someone you knew who changed (or failed to change) the course of your life. What would you say to that person if you met him or her today?

7 Think of the five things you remember best about your parents. Parent memories are, of course, some of our most powerful. Handle with care!

8 What was the best job you ever had? And the worst? Did you follow the career you wanted? Have you enjoyed your working life or are there things you would have done differently?

9 What scene from your past would you most like to visit again? If you could, would you change anything or was it so perfect that you'd like to live it all over again?

10 Think of a day from the distant past in as much detail as you possibly can. Don't just remember people and events, but conjure up memories of things, colours, textures and smells.

Be remembered

Most of this book is about how you can remember things – but what about other people's memories of you? Sometimes it's important that they should remember you. Whether you meet people in a social context or as part of your work, it's important that they go away with a good impression that will make you stand out from the crowd. When I met the girl who was to become my wife, she had a friend who would always greet me with some interesting comment she had dreamed up in advance. 'I'm going to dye my hair green', was one of her better efforts. It worked! Everyone remembered her as the girl with green hair although, as far as I remember, she never actually got round to doing the deed.

More recently, I had trouble getting the receptionist at one of my publishers to remember my name. She didn't seem to be doing it out of malice, but was just a bit dozy. It was, however, not very inspiring when she phoned through to announce my arrival by saying, 'Mister, er, urn – just a minute – what's your name again? Oh, yeah, Robert Allen's here to see you.' What to do? Simple. I offered her a lemon drop and pointed out the name on the wrapper. It was 'TREBOR' – which is 'Robert' backwards. End of problem.

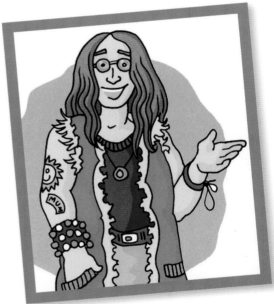

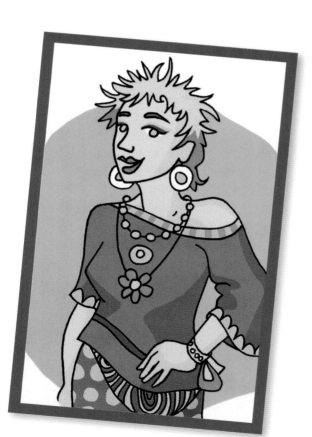

Some people have made it their business to be remembered for their eccentric appearance or behaviour. In a world where we all compete for attention, it can be important to make an impression. Even the tennis player John McEnroe's temper tantrums, widely criticized at the time, now serve him well by guaranteeing public recognition. The message? If you want to be remembered, do NOT be bland.

In my youth, I once introduced myself to a girl I fancied by writing my name on the inside of her forearm with the tip of my finger. That worked, too!

It's equally important not to be remembered for the wrong reasons. Once people know and like you they'll happily overlook all sorts of mistakes. But when you meet people for the first time, don't let them remember you for something stupid like having egg on your tie, or tripping over the carpet as you enter the office. That sort of thing will stick to you like mud.

On the other hand, some people have turned notoriety to good effect. Look at the number of actors and rock stars who have courted the public with a bad-boy or bad-girl image.

Some people like to be remembered for a trademark, such as wearing interesting ties, unusual glasses or

HYPNOPAEDIA

It was once thought that it might be possible to learn things by listening to tape recordings while sleeping. In Aldous Huxley's futuristic book *Brave New World*, the technique was the basis of all education. This was, however, one of the few predictions Huxley got wrong – but not completely wrong. If you memorize notes just before going to sleep and then put them on your bedside table (or, even better, under your pillow), it really does help to make you remember them.

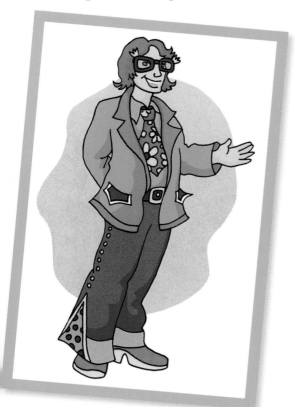

colourful clothes. This certainly works but can fall flat if it is the most interesting thing about you. A nice smile is worth cultivating because that always sticks in the memory. Having something interesting to say is good, though it is important not to sound like a Smart Alec. A colleague of mine is noted for knowing everything about everything (so he thinks). People certainly remember him – and avoid him at all costs.

Son, always tell the truth. Then you'll never have to remember what you said the last time.
Sam Rayburn

I think it is all a matter of love. The more you love a memory, the stronger and stranger it is.
Vladimir Nabokov

Memory and age

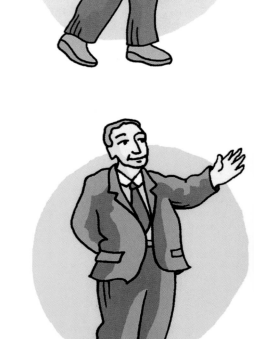

In the West, we expect that as we grow older we will deteriorate. Remember William Shakespeare's view of the ages of man in his play *As You Like It?*

All the world's a stage,
And all the men and women merely players:
They have their exits and their entrances;
And one man in his time plays many parts,
His acts being seven ages. At first the infant,
Mewling and puking in the nurse's arms.
Then the whining schoolboy, with his satchel
And shining morning face, creeping like a snail
Unwillingly to school. And then the lover,
Sighing like a furnace, with a woeful ballad
Made to his mistress' eyebrow. Then a soldier,
Full of strange oaths, and bearded like the pard,
Jealous in honour, sudden and quick in quarrel,
Seeking the bubble reputation
Even in the cannon's mouth. And then the justice
In fair round belly, with good capon lin'd,
With eyes severe and beard of formal cut,
Full of wise saws; and modern instances
And so he plays his part. The sixth age shifts
Into the lean and slipper'd pantaloon,
With spectacles on nose and pouch on side,
His youthful hose, well sav'd, a world too wide,
For his shrunk shank, and his big manly voice,
Turning again towards childish treble, pipes
And whistles in his sound. Last scene of all,
That ends this strange eventful history,
Is second childishness and mere oblivion,
Sans teeth, sans eyes, sans taste, sans everything.

Well, thanks Will, but no thanks. The Eastern view is quite the opposite. Old people are honoured and respected for their great learning and wisdom. For this reason, people have a remarkable habit of doing just what is expected of them and so there are plenty of elderly people who continue to lead active, useful lives with most of their faculties intact.

In the West we are just catching on to the idea that you don't have to grow old in the way that our parents did. This

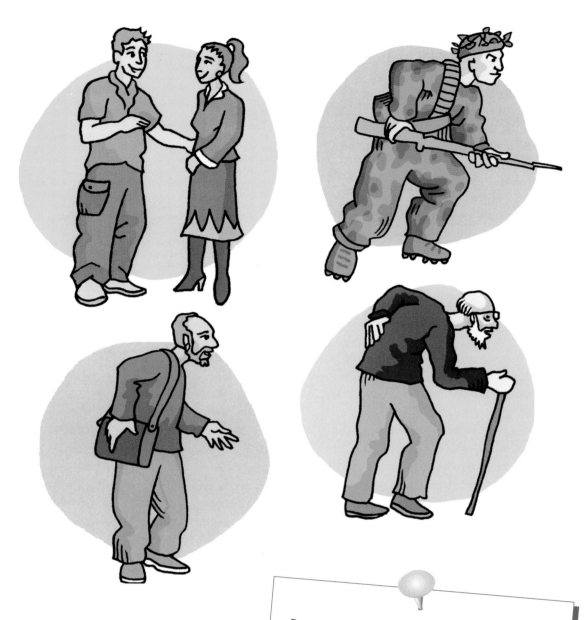

is partly a matter of mental attitude and partly due to advances in medical science. It means that you don't have to let your memory go if you don't want to. It used to be said that, as we age, our long-term memory improves (we get to bore everyone with tales of the good old days) but our short-term memory becomes unreliable. But, remember what we said at the beginning of the book: memory is a muscle – you must use it or lose it.

Drugs, alcohol and memory do not mix. This should be obvious, but after a few drinks, you may think that your understanding has miraculously improved and that you are giving the person you're talking to 100 per cent of your attention – but this is an illusion. Anything that happens when you are drunk is quite likely to be forgotten, no matter how important it is.

Open sesame!

Passwords are a plague of modern life. Most of us can't get through a single day without using them. The trouble is that you accumulate so many, it is easy to forget them. That's why just about every website you ever visit has a link marked 'Lost your password?'.

Don't you just hate passwords? How many do you have? I've got dozens of the wretched things – my e-mail accounts, my bank, various websites I visit, my cash card, passwords to get me into buildings I visit regularly – it just goes on and on. Most people get so overwhelmed by the sheer number of passwords they are expected to remember that they do some stupid things. The first one is to write all their passwords down. Don't do it! The second is to use really easy passwords. They use their name, birthday, or the registration number of their car. The whole point of a password is that it should be easy to remember but impossible for anyone else to guess.

I used to work with a bunch of extremely bright but emotionally volatile kids. One of their pastimes was to try to crack my e-mail password so that they could get in and delete my account. Little dears! I used 'OZYMANDIAS' as my password (it's the title of a poem I'd learnt at school) and, bright as my young friends undoubtedly were, not one of them ever got the password. I don't use that particular password any more, so if you want it, it's yours.

The best passwords, however, use a mixture of letters and numbers. The reason is that if you use a word on its own, a would-be hacker might just use his computer to throw the entire dictionary at your password until he finds the right word.

When I gave up 'OZYMANDIAS', I fell back on the old address password, and for a while I used 'DAIRY1953'. Now, if you were a private detective of extraordinary skill, you might guess that I once lived in an Edinburgh street called Dairy and my family moved there in 1953. But I've had loads of different addresses since then, so your chances of picking the right one are negligible. The point is that the name and number mean a lot to me, they are two of my oldest memories, but they mean nothing to anyone else. (And, of course, I've lied to you about the street, the number and the city. Just how daft do you think I am?)

*The memory has so little talent for photography.
It likes to paint pictures. Experience is not laid away in it
like a snapshot to be withdrawn at will but is returned to us
as a portrait painted in our own psychic colours, its form
and pattern structured on that of our life.*
Lillian Smith, *The Journey*

*Some memories are realities, and are better than
anything that can ever happen to one again.*
Willa Cather, *My Antonia*

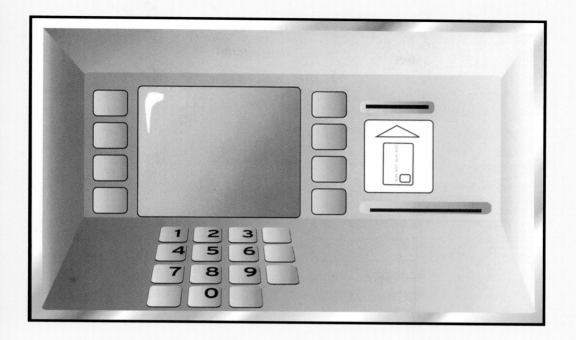

☆ Never choose anything obvious (like your name, for example).

☆ Try to use things that only you will know (your mother's maiden name is a favourite and is hard to guess).

☆ If possible, don't rely on words alone. Use a mixture of words and numbers.

☆ Don't ever write down a password anywhere. Especially not in a 'safe place'.

☆ Remember to include your passwords in your regular memory revision sessions. There are few things as aggravating as a forgotten password.

☆ Change passwords regularly.

OH, HOW, I COUNT ON YOU!

The British have a strange habit of confusing the letter 'O' with the number zero, Everyone knows that it's wrong, but they do it anyway. This has a fortunate side-effect in that it can make numbers more memorable. Turn all the zeros into little gasps of exclamation, then a rather boring telephone number like 020 7314 1400 suddenly becomes much more exciting – oh! 2 oh! 7314 14 oh! oh!

Things that help

Whatever techniques you favour, there are a number of things you can do to make memorization more effective. You should always do all of these things if you want to get the very best results. You'll hear me repeat these tips throughout the book and this is quite intentional (because repetition is a good way of making people remember).

Divide and conquer

Never try to remember whole chunks of information in one go. Break any large task into a series of smaller ones. If there are natural breaks, so much the better. See the 'Learn the kings and queens of England' on pages 92–93, where I have suggested splitting them into their royal houses for ease of recollection. This contrasts with 'Presidents of the USA', on pages 98–101, who have to be split artificially because they don't fall into neat groups.

Rest and repeat

Don't try to master something in one session. The mind is a funny thing and it goes on working even when we have apparently taken a rest. This process is very important and must be given a chance to work. Work on a memory task for no more than twenty minutes and then put it to one side. Try again the next day, and the next. You can have several tasks ongoing at the same time if you wish. You will find that by resting and revising, you will form very strong memories.

Attack from all sides

Don't always use just one method. I'll show you how to combine several methods for a much better result. If you enjoy listening most, make the Rhyme & Rhythm technique your No.1 wherever appropriate, but be sure to use other methods in addition. Tap out the rhythm with a pencil. Remember to look, look, look! Visualize what you are trying to remember. Shut your eyes and see the information in your mind's eye. Say the words out loud so that you hear yourself and learn by listening. Repeat, repeat, repeat. Do everything over and over again until you get it perfect. Repetition is not a strong method used on its own but it is highly effective if combined with others.

We seem to be going through a period of nostalgia, and everyone seems to think yesterday was better than today. 1 don't think it was, and 1 would advise you not to wait ten years before admitting today was great. If you're hung up on nostalgia, pretend today is yesterday and just go out and have one hell of a time.

Art Buchwald

Review

Review your efforts regularly. You needn't waste valuable time doing this – you can make use of odd moments such as when travelling to work or standing in the shower. These review sessions can be quite pleasurable and they will keep your memories up to date. Even the strongest memory will fade or – even worse – become unreliable if it is not refreshed from time to time.

Take your time

Do not rush memorization. Accuracy is much more important than speed. If you concentrate on accurate memorization, you will build up speed as you get more experienced – you will also be able to remember larger chunks of information at one sitting, when you have practised enough.

Work, don't worry

Getting worried about remembering things is the worst thing you can do. If you work steadily, you will build confidence in your ability to remember and you won't need to worry. If you are revising for an exam, start early. It is much easier to learn material reliably if you can work at it over a period of weeks and months rather than trying to cram it all in at the last minute.

Find a bit of time that is underused (such as waiting in heavy traffic) and make that your regular memory review spot.
It will while away a boring part of your day and add something useful to your life.

What to remember?

Theoretically, there is no limit to what you can remember. Your brain has huge amounts of spare capacity that you can fill up with whatever takes your fancy. There is no problem about your ability to remember whatever you want. But there are a couple of dangers lurking. The first is that you may commit stuff to memory using a strong memory glue and then the information rapidly becomes superfluous to requirements and can be discarded. The second is that there is no way of forgetting intentionally. Once something has been memorized, it will stay with you. Of course, if you don't review it regularly it will eventually fade – probably.

The trouble is that memory is tricky and you can never be quite sure when some old memory will suddenly pop into your consciousness. If you make the mistake, in a first flush of enthusiasm, of trying to memorize *everything*, you might find that your mind gets a bit clogged up with trash. Although, as I have pointed out,

the human mind is not at all like a computer, we might usefully draw an analogy with computer's hard drive. You know how, when you first buy the thing, everything is beautifully orderly and you can find anything you want immediately? Then, after a while, you load more and more junk on until, even though there is plenty of space left, the system slows down because it has to deal with all the detritus littering your hard drive.

Really useful things to memorize:

☆ **Personal data – names, addresses, telephone numbers, passwords**

These are always worth committing to memory because a lost address book can reduce your life to a shambles in no time. Although there is inevitably a certain amount of coming and going among your friends and acquaintances, there is always a hard core of people whose details you will need to have to hand.

☆ **Exam data**

There is some stuff that we are condemned to remember for life, whether we like it or not. It would be nice to use a weak memory glue so that we could dump all this stuff when the exam season is over but, sadly, that won't get the results we need. So, if

> Think of your memory as a library. Try to keep it orderly, and the shelves well stocked but not overloaded.

Invention, strictly speaking, is little more than a new combination of those images which have been previously gathered and deposited in the MEMORY; nothing can come from nothing.

Sir Joshua Reynolds

you want to pass exams, you need to use a strong glue and fix those physics formulae, historical dates and grammatical terms for ever.

☆ Professional data

In most jobs, and certainly in all professions, there is a certain amount of information that you need to keep, even though you might not need to refer to it every day, and this can be committed to memory profitably.

☆ Evidence

There is one area where committing stuff to memory is a spectacular success, and that is the arena of argument. If you are involved in any sort of dispute, whether it is at a small, local level, or in the wilder world of public affairs, there is no substitute for: having all the facts at the tips of your fingers. Many people argue on the basis of unsubstantiated opinion, and this is quite worthless. Why should your opinion carry any more weight than anyone else's? What you need, if you want to punch above your weight, is real evidence and the facts and figures to back it up.

☆ Cultural artefacts

Our minds operate like a garden compost heap. All sorts of rubbish goes in and is rotted down until it produces something wonderful and nourishing from which great ideas grow. A large part of this process happens naturally but, if you want to give it a helping hand, it is quite useful to have a store of cultural artefacts (poems, stories, odd and interesting bits of information) that will nourish your mind and increase your creative flow. Once again, what you memorize is absolutely up to you. But try to introduce a sense of purpose and a bit of structure into your memorization and you will find it much more effective.

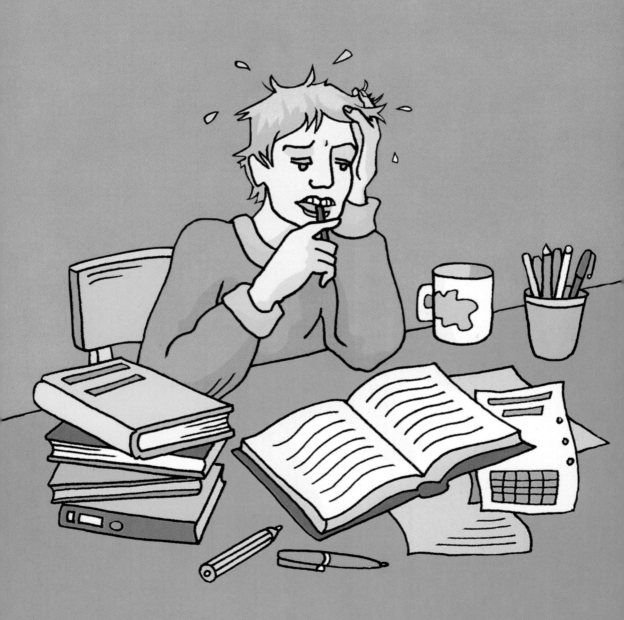

Memory Tasks

The purpose of this section is to help you test the new memory skills you have acquired. There are a variety of tasks that cover different sorts of memory and require different approaches. After describing each task, I have set out some ways in which you might attempt it. These are only *suggestions*. There is no right way to memorize, there is only the right way *for you*. Any method that works for you, no matter how eccentric it might seem to others, is OK because it works. In memory, results are all that count. Anything that helps you to attain 100 per cent accuracy and to retain important information over long periods of time, is a good method.

The tasks in this section are designed to challenge your new-found memory skills in numerous ways. There is no need to do them all in one go (in fact, such a rush of enthusiasm would do you very little good). Instead, you should take a measured approach and work at one task until you are really happy that you have learned the lessons it has to teach. Don't be put off if the knowledge imparted by a particular task is not especially useful to you. The tests are there to train you in memory methods which, eventually, you will be able to apply to tasks that are of specific importance to your own life. Don't try to memorize too quickly. Accuracy is the vital thing and speed will come in good time.

When you are confident in your new abilities go to the Mammoth Memory Test on page 139 to see just how well your memory works.

Don't try to memorize too quickly.

Never try to learn too much at once.

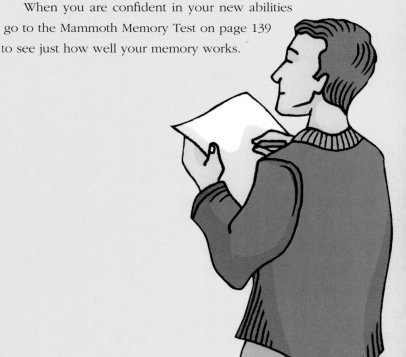

LONG-TERM MEMORY TASK
The alphabet backwards

TIME: **3 minutes** LEVEL: **Easy**

All you have to do is memorize the alphabet backwards. You may well have done this already when you were a kid, but can you do it right now without thinking? Probably not. Three minutes from now you'll be able to do it again.

Instructions

1 Start by looking at the alphabet below in this unfamiliar guise.

2 Set the whole thing to a well-known tune, such as *Twinkle, Twinkle Little Star*. If the tune doesn't quite fit the letters, that's a good thing because the glitch will make the whole task even more memorable.

Retest: Repeat the exercise later in the day and rehearse it daily for a week, then include it in your regular review sessions.

Z Y X W
R Q P O
I H G F E

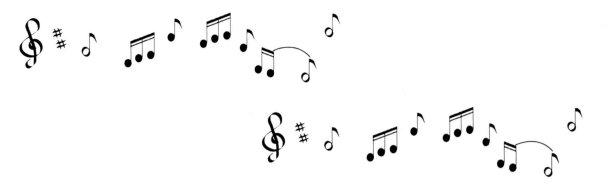

Remember this!

Divide and conquer. Don't try to learn the whole thing at one go, but break it into chunks. Keep repeating the song and add another chunk after every couple of repetitions. You should have the whole thing off pat in about fifteen minutes.

V U T S

N M L K J

D C B A

LONG-TERM MEMORY TASK

The NATO phonetic alphabet

TIME: **10 minutes** LEVEL: **Easy**

The armed forces, police, emergency services, air traffic control and numerous other bodies use the phonetic alphabet and numbers when spelling things out over the airwaves. It is international, whether you are talking to someone in India, Italy, Japan or New Jersey, it is always understood. This makes it quite a useful thing to learn.

Instructions

Here we'll use a bit of repetition, a bit of 'divide and conquer', and a kinaesthetic method.

1 Split the alphabet into five chunks of four letters (you can learn the numbers, which are very easy, separately) Yankee and Zulu, of course, are left as a group of two.
2 Now, as you repeat them to yourself, write them down each time. Alternatively, you could write them down just once and tap each word with a pencil as you say it, but I would recommend the extra effort of writing them during each repetition.
3 Now, introduce a bit of rhythm into your recitation – try slow, slow, quick, quick, slow.
4 Finally, when you are confident that you have it all well memorized, get someone to test you.

Retest: Revise daily for a week, and then from time to time.

0 Zero
1 Wun
2 Too
3 Three
4 Fower
5 Fife
6 Six
7 Seven
8 Ait
9 Niner

. Decimal
. stop

A Alpha
B Bravo
C Charlie
D Delta
E Echo
F Foxtrot
G Golf
H Hotel
I India
J Juliet
K Kilo
L Lima
M Mike

N November
O Oscar
P Papa
Q Quebec
R Romeo
S Sierra
T Tango
U Uniform
V Victor
W Whisky
X X-ray
Y Yankee
Z Zulu

LONG-TERM MEMORY TASK

Awkward spellings

TIME: **20 minutes** LEVEL: **Easy**

When I taught my daughter to spell, I didn't know as much about memory as I do now, and so I used the repetition method. Result? Each week she got top marks in the spelling test but a week later she'd forgotten the previous week's lesson completely. There are much better ways to learn to spell. Here are some suggestions on how to learn and remember correct spellings, and a list of words to learn.

☆ **Try mnemonics. For example, 'Never Eat Cake Eat Salmon Sandwiches And Remain Young' will give you the spelling of NECESSARY.**

☆ **I found this method in Roald Dahl's book *Matilda*. If you want to learn RECEIVE you learn it as: Mrs R, Mrs E, Mrs CEI, Mrs V, Mrs E.**

☆ **Divide and Conquer. If you want to learn CONSCIENTIOUS, you can split it into CON, SCI, ENT, IOUS.**

☆ **Try splitting words into bits that make some sort of bizarre sense. I had trouble with TOMORROW until I memorized it as TOM OR ROW.**

☆ **Say words to yourself exactly as they are spelled. If you want to learn RECEIPT, learn to say it as REKEP-IT. Learn ANCIENT by calling it AN-KEE-ENT. (OK, theoretically you might end up putting a K in ancient, but you're much brighter than that, aren't you?)**

Below you will find a list of the most commonly misspelled words. Go through it and cross off the ones (there will probably be many) that you can spell with confidence. Then use the methods outlined above to learn the others.

A	acceptance	adequate	aggressive	amateur
aardvark	accessible	adhesive	agitate	ambidextrous
abbreviate	accidentally	adieu	aisle	amoeba
abscond	accommodate	adjacency	alchemy	amphibian
absorbent	acoustic	adversary	algae	amphitheatre
abundant	acquiesce	aerator	align	ancestor
abysmal	acquit	aerial	allege	ancillary
academy	across	aesthetic	allegiance	anecdote
accappella	acrylic	afterwards	allowance	aneurysm
acceptable	actor	against	almond	annihilate
acceptably	actually	aggravate	already	anniversary

annoyance
annoyed
anomalous
anomaly
anonymous
antecedent
anxiety
anxious
apart
apartheid
apathetic
apologize
apostrophe
apparatus
appliqué
armament
armistice
asbestos
asphalt
assimilate
asterisk
asthma
asymmetric
aurora
austere
Australia
autumn
auxiliary

B
bankruptcy
banquet
bargain
baroque
bayonet
bayou
bazaar
beautiful
because
behaviour
beige
believe
benefit
beret

bestiary
biased
bicycle
biscuit
bivouac
bizarre
blossom
bouquet
bourgeoisie
boutique
boycott
broccoli
brochure
brogue
bruise
buoy
buoyant
bureau
bureaucratic
business

C
cabinet
Caesar
café
caffeine
calf
callous
callus
calves
camouflage
campaign
candidate
canoe
cantaloupe
captain
captor
cartilage
cataclysm
category
caterpillar
cauliflower
cavern
cease

celebration
cello
cemetery
chameleon
champagne
chandelier
charisma
chartreuse
chassis
chimney
chisel
chocolate
choir
cholera
chorale
choreograph
chronicle
chronological
chutzpah
circuit
circumstance
cliché
coalesce
coercion
cognac
cognizant
cohabiting
coiffure
collaboration
colleague
collegiate
cologne
commitment
compass
concatenate
conceit
connotation
conquer
conscious
consider
consistent
corduroy
correlate
corrugated

coup
couple
courage
course
courteous
coyote
creator
creche
creosote
cretaceous
critique
crocodile
croquet
crotch
crucifixion
cuckoo
cuisine
cul-de-sac
culottes
cupboard
curmudgeon
curriculum
czar

D
daiquiri
Dalmatian
damn
dearth
debris
debut
definable
delimiter
dependency
description
desiccation
desirable
diamond
diarrhoea
dilate
dilemma
diphtheria
diphthong
dirigible

disappointed
disciple
disgusting
dissection
dissemination
dissertation
dissipate
double
doubly
doubt
dropping
drought
dumb
dungeon
dying

E
easy
eavesdrop
ecstasy
editing
elementary
embankment
encompass
endeavour
endure
ensued
enthusiastic
entrance
entrepreneur
estuary
etiquette
eulogy
eunuch
euphoric
euthanasia
exaggerate
excellent
excerpt
excitement
explanation
extension
extraordinary

F

façade
facetious
farce
fascinate
fasten
fastened
feasible
February
fertile
feud
flood
flotation
fluorescent
forehead
foreign
forfeit
forty
fuchsia
fulfil
funeral
futile

G

gaiety
gauge
geisha
genealogy
generally
genuine
geyser
ghastly
ghost
ghoul
gingham
glycerine
gourd
government
governor
grammar
granary
grandiose
guerrilla
guess

guillotine
guitar
gymnast

H

haemorrhage
hallelujah
heifer
height
heinous
heuristic
hiatus
hierarchy
history
homage
horrible
hors d'oeuvre
hydraulics
hygienic
hymn

I

icicle
idiosyncrasy
illegal
illegitimate
illustrate
imbalance
immediately
immense
impressed
impugn
inception
inheritance
instantiation
instrument
intent
interfere
interference
interpret
interpretation
interrupt
intrigue
intuitive

invocation
invoke
isthmus

J

jagged
jalousie
jealous
jealousy
jeopardize
jewel
journal
journey

K

kaleidoscope
kayak
ketchup
khaki
kibbutz
kiosk
knife
knowledge
knowledgeable

L

label
labyrinth
lacquer
laid
lasagne
legionnaire
legitimacy
legitimate
leisure
lenient
light
lightning
likelihood
limousine
lingerie
liquor
literature
llama

luau
luggage
luscious

M

maelstrom
maestro
maintain
maintenance
malice
malicious
mannequin
manoeuvre
marquee
marriage
marshmallow
martyr
masochist
matinee
mausoleum
mayonnaise
medieval
millennium
miniature
minuscule
miscellaneous
mischievous
missile
misspell
moccasin
months
morgue
mortgage
mosquito
muscle
myrrh
mystic
mystique

N

naive
naivety
nasturtium
nauseous

necessarily
necessary
neighbour
neither
neural
niche
night
ninety
noticeable
noxious
nuance
nuisance
nutritious
nymph

O

obelisk
obey
oblique
occasion
occurred
odyssey
officially
often
omelette
onomatopoeia
opaque
opinion
opportunity
oracle
orang-utan
orchestrate
orchid
oregano
oscillate
oscilloscope
ostrich
ovation
overwhelm

P

pageant
paradigm
parallel

parameter
paraphernalia
parliament
parquet
participate
peace
peignoir
penitentiary
people
perform
perhaps
perimeter
persistence
persistent
pertain
pertinent
pewter
phlegm
piedmont
plagiarism
plagiarize
plague
plaid
plaque
pollinate
possession
postpone
potpourri
precede
precious
precursor
Presbyterian
presence
prestigious
primitive
privilege
prolix
pronunciation
proprietary
proprietor
protein
protocol
pseudonym
ptarmigan

pterodactyl
pumpkin
pursue
pylon
Pyrrhic

Q

quadruple
questionnaire
queue
quiche

R

rabbit
radius
rapport
raspberry
rather
realm
receipt
receive
recipe
recommend
reconnaissance
recurrence
regardless
rehearsal
reindeer
relief
religion
remain
renaissance
rendezvous
repertoire
replenish
reservoir
responsibility
responsible
rhythm
ricochet
riddled
ridiculous

S

saboteur
saccharin
safety
salmon
sandwich
satellite
savvy
scaffolding
scenario
schizophrenic
scissors
scourge
scythe
segue
seismograph
seizure
sense
sensible
separate
sepulchral
sergeant
serious
severe
sherbet
should
shoulder
siege
sienna
sleuth
solder
subpoena
subtle
successfully
supplement
suppress
surgeon
suspicion
sword
syllable
syllabus
synagogue
synonymous
syringe

T

tarpaulin
technician
technique
tedious
temporary
temptation
tendency
terrain
terrible
terrific
Teutonic
their
theorem
theory
therapeutic
there
thereby
thief
thieves
thirtieth
thistle
thought
threshold
tomato
tomatoes
tongue
torque
tortellini
tortoise
toucan
tournament
transcend
transition
transmission
trauma
triathlon
tries
trigonometric
trinket
troubadour
trudging
true
truly

U

unanimous
unduly
usability
useful

V

vacuum
variant
variation
vaudeville
vegetarian
vehement
vehicle
veterinarian
vigilante
vignette
vinaigrette
vinegar
vinyl

W

weasel
weird
wherever
whisper
whistle
wholly
wildebeest
withdrawal
would
wrestle
writable

Y

yacht
yeoman

Z

zealot
zephyr
zinc
zucchini

VISUAL MEMORY TASK

Playing cards

TIME: **5 mins** LEVEL: **Easy**

Memorizing playing cards is one of those things that trick memorizers do. They even have championships to see who can memorize the most cards in the shortest time. So why is it included here? Well, performed in strict moderation, it is an exercise that will help strengthen your visual memory

Instructions

Opposite you'll see pictures of 25 cards in five rows of five. First, learn the cards in the order given (left to right, top to bottom). When you are confident of being able to do it in order, it is time to try recalling them at random. When you have completed the test with the cards I have given you, work with arrangements of your own.

Try one (or all) of the methods described opposite to memorize the cards. Now, cover the page and test yourself.

1 Which card is in the top right-hand corner?
2 Which card is at the bottom of the middle column?
3 What is to the right of the 4 of Hearts?
4 What is below the Jack of Clubs?
5 What comes below the 10 of Clubs?
6 Is the 3 of Spades on the diagram?
7 What comes two places above the 4 of Hearts?
8 Which two cards flank the 9 of Hearts?
9 What is at the top of the column that has the 3 of Diamonds at the bottom?
10 What is at the extreme right of the row that has the Jack of Clubs on the left?
11 What comes below the King of Spades?

12 Which column is headed by the Ace of Hearts?
13 Where is the Queen of Diamonds?
14 Where is the Ace of Clubs?
15 What is at the bottom of the column headed by the 2 of Clubs?

How to do it

☆ Don't just rely on the pictures in the book, but get out your own cards and *handle* them as you memorize. Touching the cards is a very important part of the process.

☆ If you have a good visual memory (and many people don't), you could try to visualize the cards laid out on an imaginary table in your head. Alternatively, it might be more fun, and more effective, to visualize the cards as people. Instead of thinking 'King of Hearts' why not think of someone you know dressed as a king and wearing a heart badge? Queen of Hearts – why not J-Lo? For the knaves, you can supply politicians of your choice. Aces could be represented by sports stars, and so on. Use your imagination and have fun.

☆ If you are a Listener (see page 13), you should recite the names of the cards to yourself. Remember that sing-song rhythm that you used to chant at school? Well, that is *just* the one you need – something nice and catchy that will stick in the memory.

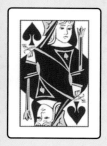   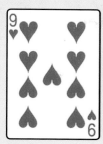 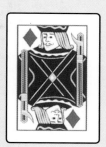

 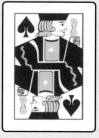 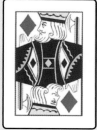  

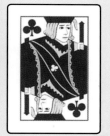 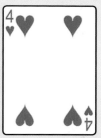 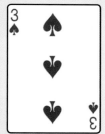  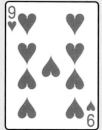

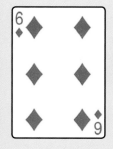 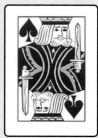 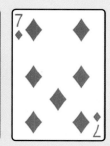 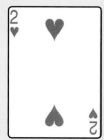 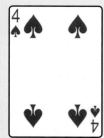

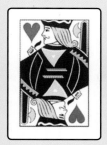 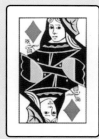 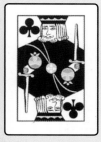 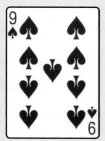 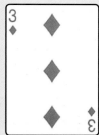

I'm sorry, I've forgotten your name

TIME: **5 minutes** LEVEL: **Easy**

It's embarrassing to forget people's names because it implies that they aren't important to you. Opposite you'll find a group of twelve faces and your task for today is to remember them. We have deliberately not put names under the faces because, in real life, how often does that happen? Only at conferences where people wear badges. The people are (from left to right and top to bottom):

Row 1 Wendy Dear, Tom Armstrong, April McDonald

Row 2 Carmen Garcia, Jim Russell, Kelly Drummond

Row 3 Allen Levi, Janie Wilderspin, Frank Wright

Row 4 Ivana Lloyd, Miles Hill, Hayley Kellow

Instructions

Start with the faces. Most people have something about their features that allows you to give them a nickname. The name can be as funny as you like (the funnier the better, in fact). Don't worry about being cruel – it's your own private name and you needn't confide it to anyone else. Once you know that, for example, Jim Russell has a rather prominent nose, you can call him Beaky and you'll always remember him like that.

Now, to remember the names. You only need one memorable feature in each name. For example, once you remember that Mr Armstrong has a Strong Arm, you'll easily attach the name Tom to the memory. Wendy Dear can be transformed into the more affectionate Dear Wendy. April McDonald? How about visualizing eating a burger on a showery day? Carmen is an easy name to remember because of the opera (just think about toreadors). Is Kelly Drummond a drummer? Can Allen (think of Woody) Levitate? Is Janie wild and in a spin? Frank Wright, of course reminds you of Frank Lloyd Wright (and the Paul Simon song). Ivana is, of course, terrible and Miles Hill lives at the top of a very long rise. As for Hayley Kellow; she's no problem. I have a friend called Kellow and people always either say, 'Hello, Kellow' or they call her 'Cornflake' (after Kellogg's cornflakes).

Remember this!

Is this all silly and immature? Excellent! The sillier and more childish you can be, the more likely you are to remember.

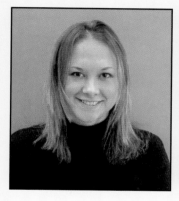
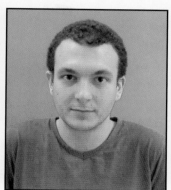
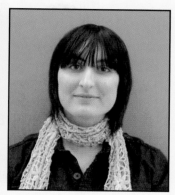

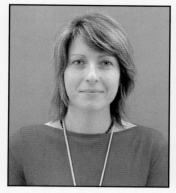
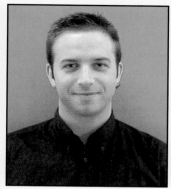
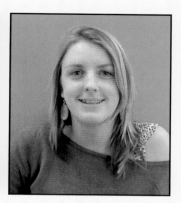

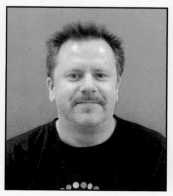
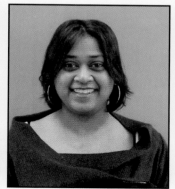
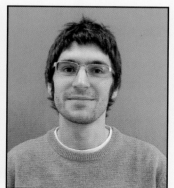

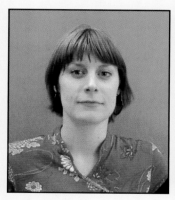
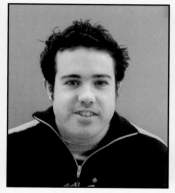
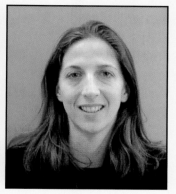

SHORT-TERM MEMORY TASK
Dates

TIME: **30 minutes** LEVEL: **Medium**

At one time, learning history was all about dates. Nowadays that is thought unnecessary (and so kids know what happened and maybe even why it happened, but don't have the slightest idea when). If you just want to learn the years in which things happened, one way to do it is to regard the dates as times from a 24-hour clock. Then, for example, the signing of Magna Carta can be remembered as 12.15 p.m. (just in time for lunch!).

Here are 30 dates to memorize (you can, of course, choose your own):

1895: Juan Peron (President of Argentina 1946–55) born.

1941: Jesse Jackson, American civic leader and clergyman, born.

1949: Sigourney Weaver, American actress, born.

1787: William Herschel discovers that the planet Uranus has moons.

1831: HMS Beagle, with Charles Darwin on board, sets sail on its world voyage.

1927: Leon Trotsky expelled from the Communist Party.

1994: Nelson Mandela sworn in as the President of South Africa.

1958: Hawaii becomes the 50th state of the United States of America.

1950: Edgar Rice Burroughs, the American novelist, author of the *Tarzan* books, dies.

1608: Quebec, Canada founded by Samuel Champlain.

1863: Battle of Gettysburg, during the American Civil War, ends.

1928: First colour TV transmission, made by John Logie Baird.

1833: Alfred Nobel, Swedish inventor of dynamite, born.

1908: First Model T Ford produced in Detroit.

1949: The People's Republic of China created.

1971: Disneyworld opens in Orlando, Florida.

1920: Panama Canal opened by the President of America, Woodrow Wilson.

1823: The waterproof material for raincoats patented by Charles Macintosh.

1944: Iceland becomes an independent republic.

1946: War crime trial of Emperor Hirohito of Japan begins.

1967: China explodes its first H-bomb.

1792: France becomes a republic, abolishing its monarchy.

1915: Stonehenge sold at auction for £6,600.

1917: Latvia proclaims independence.

1622: Papal Chancery adopts January as beginning of the year.

1660: Englishman Samuel Pepys begins his famous diary.

1863: Emancipation Proclamation (ending slavery) issued by General Abraham Lincoln.

1939: General Franco conquers Barcelona.

1945: Soviet forces reach Auschwitz concentration camp.

1849: Safety pin patented in USA.

Instructions

Sort all the events into chronological order. Why didn't I do it for you? Because sorting them out for yourself is the start of the learning process. Next, draw a timeline to scale about 7 cm (3 inches), for each hundred years) and mark the dates on it. When you've done it once, put it to one side and, on a clean sheet of paper, try redrawing it from memory. As you draw your timeline, read it out to yourself.

Some people like to remember numbers by their shapes (so 1 is a stick, 0 is a ball, 8 is a fat lady, 2 is a duck, and so on). Then you make up stories that put the shapes together. I never have the patience for this, but if it works for you don't let me stand in your way.

Close your eyes and imagine that you are carving your timeline in stone (you can even act out hammering a chisel into stone if it helps).

As always, learn the list a bit at a time and keep reviewing it.

Now try this test

1 When did the Battle of Gettysburg end?
2 When was the first Model T Ford produced?
3 When did Franco conquer Barcelona?
4 When was the first colour TV transmission?
5 When did Hawaii become the 50th state of the USA?
6 When did HMS *Beagle* set sail?
7 When did China explode its first H-bomb?
8 When did Samuel Pepys start to write his diary?
9 What major event occurred in South Africa in 1994?
10 When did Charles Macintosh patent his waterproof raincoat material?
11 When did Latvia become independent?
12 When did the Soviets liberate Auschwitz?
13 What happened in Barcelona in 1939?
14 When was Trotsky expelled from the Communist Party?
15 When was Stonehenge sold at auction and how much did it fetch?

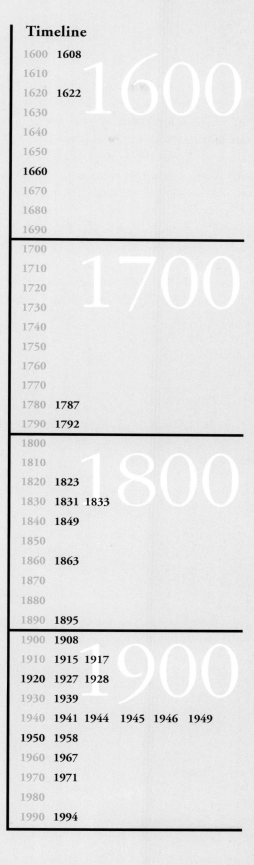

Timeline

1600	**1608**
1610	
1620	**1622**
1630	
1640	
1650	
1660	
1670	
1680	
1690	
1700	
1710	
1720	
1730	
1740	
1750	
1760	
1770	
1780	**1787**
1790	**1792**
1800	
1810	
1820	**1823**
1830	**1831 1833**
1840	**1849**
1850	
1860	**1863**
1870	
1880	
1890	**1895**
1900	**1908**
1910	**1915 1917**
1920	**1927 1928**
1930	**1939**
1940	**1941 1944 1945 1946 1949**
1950	**1958**
1960	**1967**
1970	**1971**
1980	
1990	**1994**

LONG-TERM MEMORY TASK

Half a pound of tuppenny rice

TIME: **10 minutes** LEVEL: **Easy**

Ever got to the supermarket and found that you've forgotten your shopping list? Aaaaagh! Few things are more frustrating. If your house is like ours, one person makes the shopping list and everyone else yells out the things that they want, so you end up with a mass of items in no particular order. It is helpful to convert this list into a form that can be remembered more easily, then if you forget your list, it should not pose such a problem!

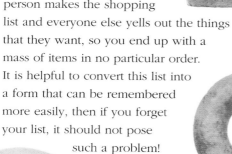

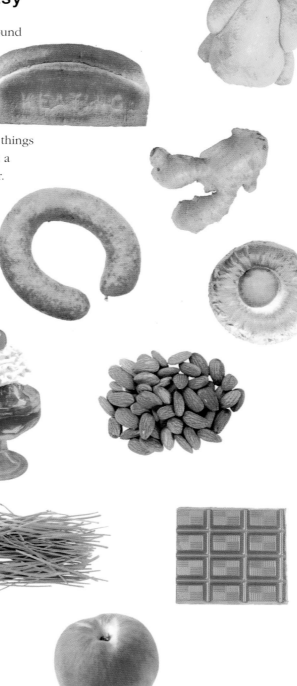

Instructions

In our house, my wife has a clever trick. She always takes the same route around the supermarket. This forms a little ritual and, as we have seen elsewhere, ritual is an excellent memory aid. So, let's write down all the items in a way that makes some sort of logistical sense:

★ Cheese and desserts are near to each other.
★ Mushrooms, bell peppers, lettuce, fresh herbs are near the entrance.
★ Ginger is close to peaches.
★ Salami, chicken and fish aren't far apart.
★ Chilli powder is opposite the cans of spaghetti and noodles.
★ Eggs are on their own.
★ Crackers are just before pastries and loaves, which are together.
★ Nachos and almonds can be found close together.
★ Chocolate is on its own.
★ Razors are near the checkout.

Draw your own plan of the supermarket (it needn't be all that accurate), write the names of the items on slips of paper and put them face down in the right places. Now practise picking them up and naming the items *before* you turn the slips over. After a few attempts, you should start to get it right.

The beauty of this system is that once you have the basic scheme in your mind, you can easily make a few mental notes about additions and deletions. A regular route also helps ensure that you do not miss items that form a standard part of your shopping requirements.

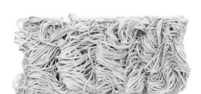

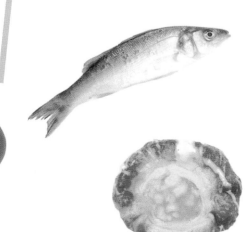

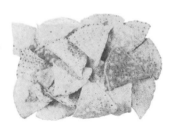

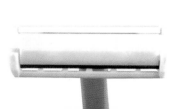

Signs of the zodiac

TIME: **15 minutes**

LEVEL: **Medium**

You can either learn the signs of the zodiac by date (which gives you a nice framework into which they fit and makes learning easier), or you can split them into elements, symbols or seasons as shown here.

Elements

FIRE	AIR
Aries	Gemini
Leo	Libra
Sagittarius	Aquarius

EARTH	WATER
Taurus	Cancer
Virgo	Scorpio
Capricorn	Pisces

Instructions

Each sign has a symbol that is traditionally associated with it. Use the symbols shown opposite as visual clues to help you remember each sign. To give you another visual clue, the symbols are depicted on a diagram showing the year as a circle, with each of the four seasons in a different colour. This should help you to fix the various symbols firmly in your memory.

Dates

Aries	March 21 – April 20
Taurus	April 21 – May 21
Gemini	May 22 – June 21
Cancer	June 22 – July 23
Leo	July 24 – August 23
Virgo	August 24– September 23
Libra	September 24 – October 23
Scorpio	October 24 – November 22
Sagittarius	November 23 – December 22
Capricorn	December 23 – January 20
Aquarius	January 21 – February 19
Pisces	February 20 – March 20

Symbols

Aries	♈	Libra	♎
Taurus	♉	Scorpio	♏
Gemini	♊	Sagittarius	♐
Cancer	♋	Capricorn	♑
Leo	♌	Aquarius	♒
Virgo	♍	Pisces	♓

Seasons

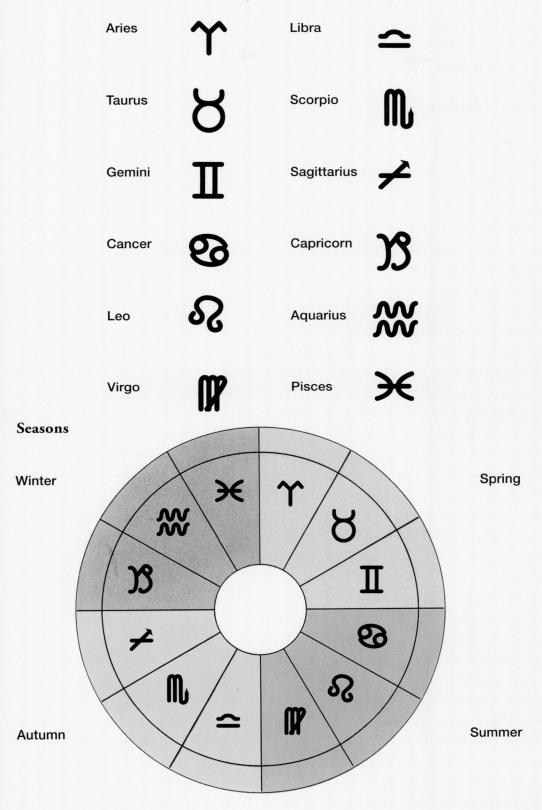

Winter

Spring

Autumn

Summer

Animal farm

TIME: **10 minutes** LEVEL: **Medium**

This is an exercise in visual memory. The picture below contains thirty animals and your job is to remember all of them. How? As usual, you must attack the problem from all angles at once.

Instructions

1   Work your way across the pictures from left to right and top to bottom.
2   Read out loud the names of the animals as you go.
3   Tap the picture of each animal as you name it.
4   Divide up the pictures into horizontal rows.
5   Frequently close your eyes and try to visualize the whole set of pictures.
6   If you want, you can make up a song to help you remember the animals in whichever order you prefer.
7   Rest for a while and then return to your memorization.
8   As with all these exercises, it is accuracy rather than speed that counts.

When you have got all the pictures fixed in your mind, cover them with a piece of paper and try to answer the following questions:

1   Which animal is to the right of the giraffe?
2   How many animals start with the letter 'C'?
3   Which animals surround the scorpion?
4   How many mammals are there on the bottom row?
5   Which animal is to the left of the owl?
6   Name all the animals that start with the letter 'L'.
7   Name all the animals on the right hand edge of the picture from top to bottom.
S   Which animal is in the bottom left hand corner?
9   How many animals start with the letter 'M'?
10 Which are the three largest animals?

Remember this!

The resting is as important as the memorization. While you rest, your mind continues to work on your task at a subconscious level.

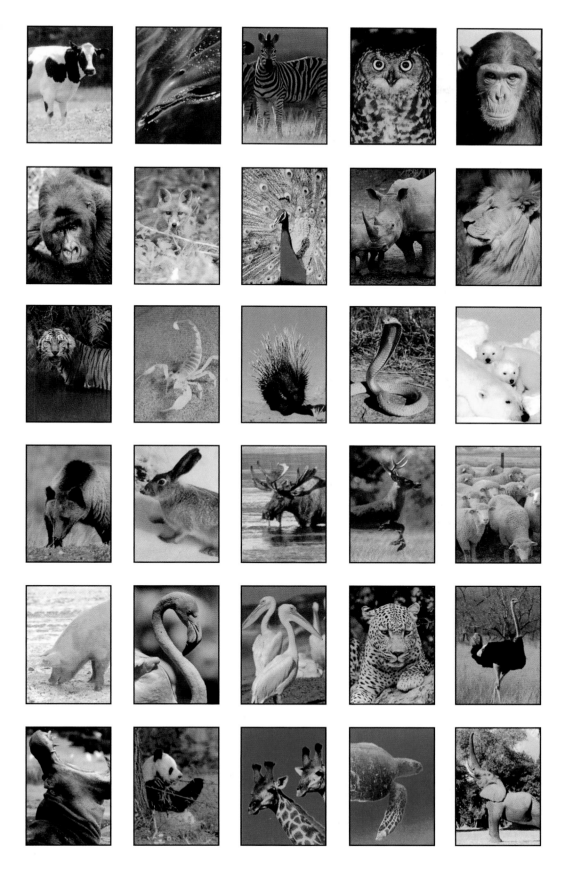

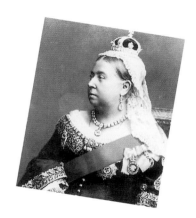

VISUAL MEMORY TASK

Learn the kings and queens of England

TIME: **1 hour** LEVEL: **Hard**

On the right you'll find the names of all the kings and queens of England since William the Conqueror. Your task is to learn them all in order. The dates of their reigns are given, but learning those is an optional extra. This is quite a major task, but there are a few things that will help you. First, there is a mnemonic that goes like this:

Willie, Willie, Harry, Steve,
Harry, Dick, John, Harry Three,
Edward One, Two and Three, Dick Two,
Henry Four, Five, Six, then who?
Edward Four, Five, Dick the Bad,
Harrys twain and Ned, the lad.
Mary, Lizzie, James the Vain,
Charlie, Charlie, James again.
William and Mary, Anne O'Gloria,
Four Georges, William and Victoria.
Edward Seven, Georgie Five,
Edward, George and Liz (alive)

This might not make much sense right now, but when you have studied the list for a while it will definitely prove helpful.

If you want to spend more time on this task, go to your local library and find pictures of these kings and queens.

Copy the images and put their names underneath to help you remember them.

I've also added a few comments that might stick in your memory. Why are we doing this? Well, because these days it's information that most people lack and it will train your memory to categorize and store quite detailed information.

Instructions

As always, I want you to attack from all angles.

1 Use the mnemonic.
2 If you have found pictures, look at them and make sure you touch them as you say the names.
3 Split the task into bits by learning the Normans, then the Plantagenets, then the Tudors, and so on.
4 Pick out kings and queens that you know about (everyone remembers Richard the Lionheart, Crookback Dick, Henry V and Henry VIII, for example), and use them as markers. You can then start filling in the gaps between them.
5 Try to build up a mental portrait gallery (visualize it in a castle if that helps). Stroll around your virtual gallery and make sure you have no blank spots on the walls.
6 Test yourself (or get someone else to test you) again and again.

NORMANS

William I	1066–1087
(William the Conqueror,	
victor of the Battle of Hastings)	
William II	1087–1100
Henry I	1100–1135
Stephen I	1135–1154
(The only Stephen)	

PLANTAGENETS

Henry II	1154–1189
Richard I	1189–1199
(Richard the Lionheart)	
John	1199–1216
(Lost his jewels in The Wash and signed	
Magna Carta)	
Henry III	1216–1272
Edward I	1272–1307
Edward II	1307–1327
Edward III	1327–1377
Richard II	1377–1399

HOUSE OF LANCASTER

Henry IV	1399–1413
Henry V	1413–1422
(Defeated the French at Agincourt)	
Henry VI	1422–1461
(Wars of the Roses)	

HOUSE OF YORK

Edward IV	1461–1483
Edward V	1483
(Deposed and killed)	
Richard III	1483–1485
(Crook-back Dick. A horse, a horse, my	
kingdom for a horse!)	

HOUSE OF TUDOR

Henry VII	1485–1509
Henry VIII	1509–1547
(Six wives: divorced, beheaded, died,	
divorced, beheaded, survived)	
Edward VI	1547–1553
Mary I	1553–1558 *(Bloody Mary)*
Elizabeth I 1558-1603	*(Good Queen Bess)*

HOUSE OF STUART

James I	1603-1625
Charles I	1625-1649
(Lost his head)	

COMMONWEALTH

Oliver Cromwell	1649–1660

HOUSE OF STUART *(continued)*

Charles II	1660–1685
James II	1685–1688
William III and Mary II	1689–1694
Anne	1702–1714

HOUSE OF HANOVER

George I	1714–1727
George II	1727–1760
George III	1760–1820
George IV	1820–1830
William IV	1830–1837
Victoria	1837–1901
Edward VII	1901–1910
George V	1910–1936
Edward VIII	1936
(Abdicated)	
George VI	1936–1952
Elizabeth II	1952–

SHORT-TERM MEMORY TASK

Café Olé!

TIME: **5 minutes** LEVEL: **Hard**

You have a part-time job waiting tables at the Café Olé. You have to learn to take customers' orders accurately without forgetting them. This is a tough job, but with a little practice, you'll get the hang of it. There are five tables in your section. Look at the picture to learn what the customers have ordered.

Instructions

1 Take the tables in an order that suits you and also put the customers into some sort of order (such as clockwise round the table, always starting in the same place).

2 Visualize a menu in your head and check off each person's choice on it.

3 Keep sweets, savouries and drinks separate in your mind.

4 Note carefully the physical appearance and dress of your customers.

5 Give people nicknames that help you to remember them.

6 As you take the orders, visualize what each person's place setting will look like when their food arrives.

7 In other exercises I have said, 'Take your time, accuracy is more important than speed.' But not this time. Who wants a slow but accurate waiter or waitress? So you must practise thinking fast and remembering orders that you have heard only once.

Now cover the illustration and try answering these questions:

1 What did the boy with the Mohican order?

2 Who had the all-day English breakfast?

3 What did the man with the beard want?

4 Which was the only table to order ice cream?

5 Who ate the fruit cake?

6 What did the girl with brown hair in the stripy green sweatshirt order?

7 Who had coffee and a scone?

8 What sort of pizza did the man with red hair want?

9 Who ordered fried chicken?

10 Who wanted fruit salad?

11 What did the guide dog have?

12 Did the woman want whipped cream with her cherry pie?

13 What did the girl with spiky hair want on her toast?

14 What did the boy want on his banana split?

15 What flavours of ice cream did the girl with blonde plaits want?

Retest: Once you can do this exercise you could make up your own and carry on practising until you get really good at it.

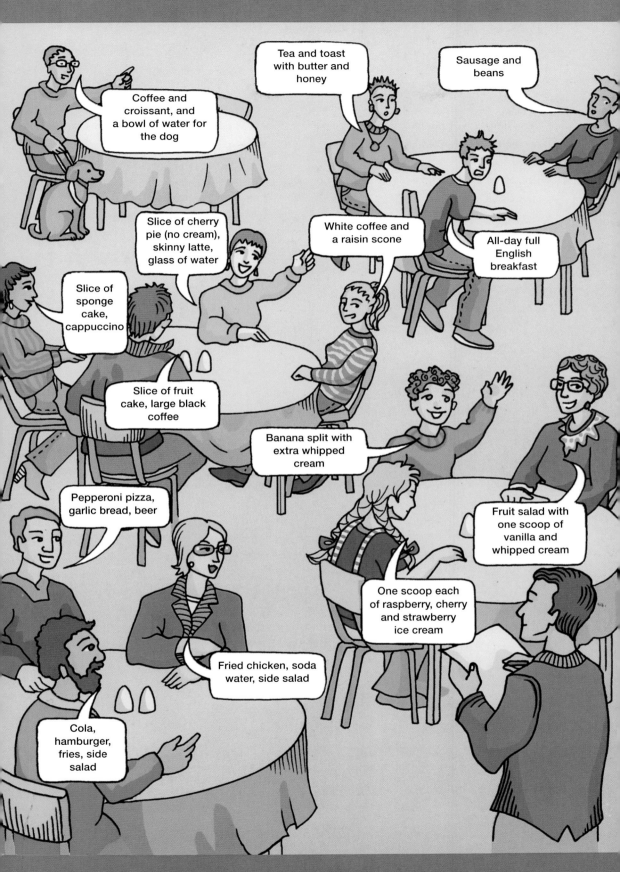

LONG-TERM MEMORY TASK
Ticket to ride
TIME: **10 minutes** LEVEL: **Hard**

Here is a railway station departure board (showing purely imaginary places) and your job is to learn it well enough to answer travellers' questions.

Instructions
What makes this a tough test is that it is hard to get to grips with so much information. What to do? This is a prime candidate for a bit of rhythm. Try reading the names to yourself in a childish, sing-song voice or, if you prefer, set them to a tune of your choice.

☆ **Tap out the rhythm as you sing.**

☆ **Visualize the board in your mind.**

☆ **Don't expect to remember everything at once. Form a basic but imperfect memory first, and then add bits to it until you have the whole thing crystal clear in your mind.**

When you feel confident that you have memorized it all, cover up the picture and try to answer these questions:

1   Which platform would you go to for the Dudstead train?
2   What time does the Harling train leave Platform 6?
3   When is the Fairfield train due to reach its destination?
4   Which train would you take to reach Goodhope?
5   Is Cranmere on the Gromby line?
6   Which station comes after Fen Grundy?
7   Which station is between Little Buckham and Grantling?
8   Which station comes after Forfar?
9   Does the Dudstead train call at Dry Hilton?
10   Does the Dudstead train reach its destination before or after the Gromby train?
11   Which station comes after Lower Morton?
12   What time does the Thorpe train arrive?
13   Which train is delayed?
14   Which train is cancelled?
15   Which is the first stop on the Thorpe line?

DEPARTURES

PLATFORM 1

FAIRFIELD

Departs	08.30
Arrives	09.15

Deacon
Abbey Morton
Lower Morton
Forfar
Bradfield
Gomers End
Hamble Point
Fairfield

PLATFORM 2

SARSTED

Departs	08.45
Arrives	09.02

Bentley
Ickleton
Cranmere
Little Spalding
Eaton Farsmworth
Sarsted

PLATFORM 3

THORPE

Departs	08.51
Arrives	09.29

Smithfield
Carlton
Goodhope
Little Buckham
Greater Buckham
Grantling
Thorpe

PLATFORM 4

DUDSTEAD

Departs	09.13
Arrives	10.16

Cancelled

Grendon
Grobley
Fen Grundy
Marsden
Jedborough
Grovely
Seven Stars
Dudstead

PLATFORM 5

GROMBY

Departs	09.27
Arrives	11.03

Flatwick
Dewenter
Dry Hilton
Gromby

PLATFORM 6

HARLING

Departs	10.12
Arrives	10.45

Charlston
Lower Sidley
Hardley
Farringthorpe
Harling

LONG-TERM MEMORY TASK

Presidents of the USA

TIME: **1 hour** LEVEL: **Hard**

Your task is to learn all the presidents of the USA, from George Washington to the present day. I have seen a number of ways recommended. One is to turn the names into a story For example, a woman washing-a-tonne (a big barrel) is watched by Adams (two men wearing nothing but fig leaves), and Jeff (who has his son with him). This does nothing for me at all and it won't work.

Another method is similar, but without the story. It involves making some amusing association with each name, thus Taylor becomes a guy stitching pants, and Lincoln drives a large automobile, and Garfield is remembered for that cat ... I don't think that's going to work either.

Instructions

Commit these American leaders to memory – there are 44 to learn, so be methodical. Let's go back to the old multiple attack method.

☆ Look at the pictures.

☆ Touch each picture as you say the name.

☆ Learn the names in blocks of a few at a time.

☆ Recite the names in some sort of rhythm. Divide the names into blocks that give you a good rhythm. The first four (Washington, Adams, Jefferson, Madison) give a really excellent rhythm but some of the others are a bit trickier.

☆ Depending on your age, you should find some of the later ones easy.

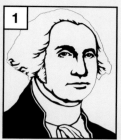

George Washington
(1732–1799)

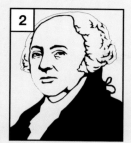

John Adams
(1735–1826)

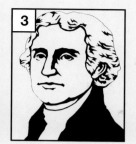

Thomas Jefferson
(1743–1826)

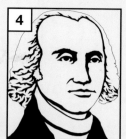

James Madison
(1751–1836)

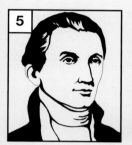

James Monroe
(1758–1831)

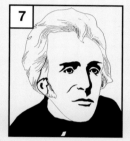

John Quincy Adams
(1767–1848)

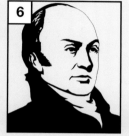

Andrew Jackson
(1767–1845)

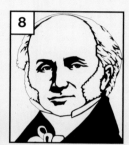

Martin van Buren
(1782–1862)

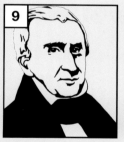

William H. Harrison
(1773–1841)

John Tyler
(1790–1862)

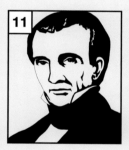

James K. Polk
(1795–1849)

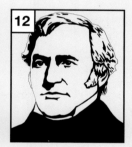

Zachary Taylor
(1784–1850)

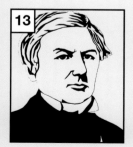

Millard Fillmore
(1800–1874)

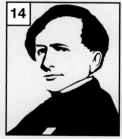

Franklin Pierce
(1804–1869)

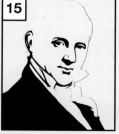

James Buchanan
(1791–1868)

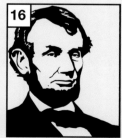

Abraham Lincoln
(1809–1865)

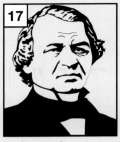

Andrew Johnson
(1808–1875)

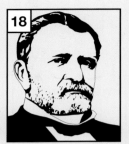

Ulysses S. Grant
(1822–1885)

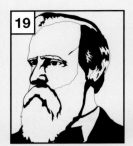

Rutherford Hayes
(1822–1893)

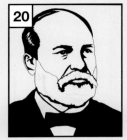

James Garfield
(1831–1881)

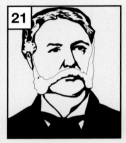

Chester Arthur
(1829–1886)

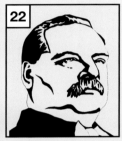

Grover Cleveland
(1837–1908)

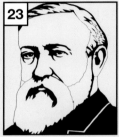

Benjamin Harrison
(1833–1901)

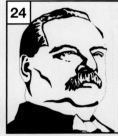

Grover Cleveland
(1837–1908)

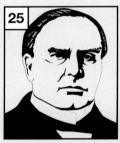

William McKinley
(1843–1901)

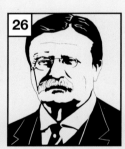

Theodore Roosevelt
(1858–1919)

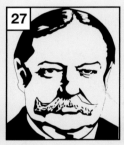

William Taft
(1857–1930)

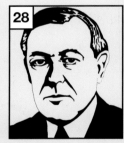

Woodrow Wilson
(1856–1924)

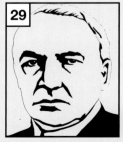

Warren Harding
(1865–1923)

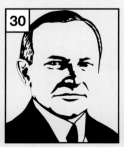

Calvin Coolidge
(1872–1933)

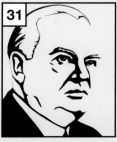

Herbert C. Hoover
(1874–1964)

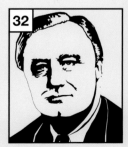

Franklin Delano
Roosevelt (1882–1945)

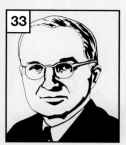

Harry S. Truman
(1884–1972)

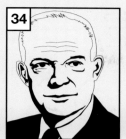

Dwight David
Eisenhower
(1890–1969)

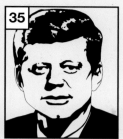

John Fitzgerald
Kennedy
(1917–1963)

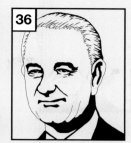

Lyndon Baines
Johnson
(1908–1973)

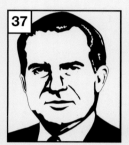

Richard Milhous
Nixon
(1913–1994)

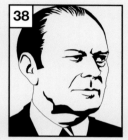

Gerald R. Ford
(1913–2006)

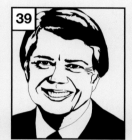

James (Jimmy)
Earl Carter Jr.
(1924–)

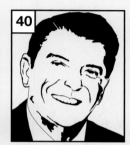

Ronald Wilson
Reagan
(1911–2004)

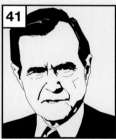

George H. W. Bush
(1924–)

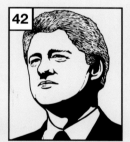

William (Bill)
Jefferson Clinton
(1946–)

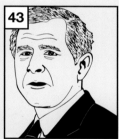

George W. Bush
(1946–)

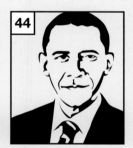

Barack Hussein
Obama
(1961–)

Learning Braille

TIME: **1 hour** LEVEL: **Hard**

Only the blind have any practical use for Braille, but don't let that put you off this exercise because it is a particularly good way of practising tactile memory. The sad truth is that most of us only use this type of memory by accident. There are some exceptions – typists, motor mechanics and surgeons spring to mind – but often this valuable ability is greatly underused.

Instructions

1 Start with the diagram opposite and try to familiarize yourself with the Braille alphabet. Just because Braille was intended to aid the blind does not mean that sighted people should fail to use all their faculties to learn it.
2 Next, make some tiles out of thin card and use glue to make the little bumps that you will learn to feel with your fingertips. Modelling glue is good for this as it will dry in little heaps without much encouragement.

3 Now you need to practise again and again until you have learnt all the letters. Start by laying them out in alphabetical order and keep handling them until you feel confident about identifying them with your eyes closed.
4 Next, try to identify random letters, again, of course, without looking.
5 When you can do this with confidence, get someone to make up words and then sentences for you to read.

You will find that with practice, you get used to using this sort of memory. It comes as a surprise to some people that tactile memory not only resides in their fingertips but in all parts of the body. If you have ever tried golf, diving, gymnastics, tai chi, or any other physical activity you will know that your body has the very useful capacity to remember how it is supposed to behave.

Braille basics

The six dots of the Braille cell are arranged and numbered like this.

The capital sign, (dot 6), placed before a letter, makes a capital letter.

The number sign (dots 3, 4, 5, 6) placed before the characters a through j, makes the numbers 1 through O. For example, 'a' preceded by the number sign is '1', 'b' is '2', and so on.

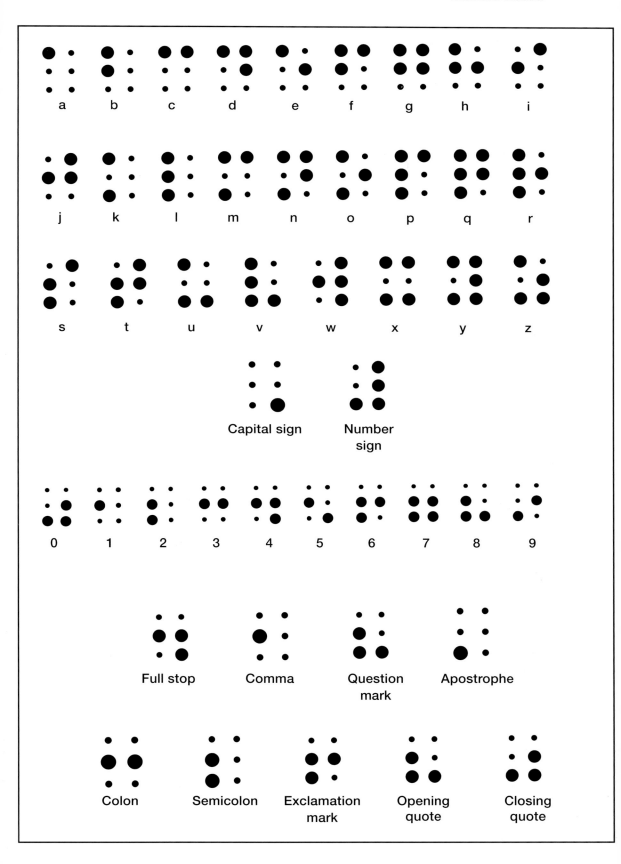

LONG-TERM MEMORY TASK
Wine bottles and their names

TIME: **1 hour** LEVEL: **Medium**

A standard bottle of wine contains 0.75 litres of liquid, but there are many variations on this basic size. Almost everyone has heard of a magnum of champagne, but did you know just how many other names there are for large bottles? No? Well, now you can learn them all. Why? There is no pressing reason why you should except that the words are fun and, who knows, one day you may be rich enough to afford a Melchior of champagne, and wouldn't it be just be your luck if you didn't know what to ask for?

The chart gives the names of 14 different bottle sizes, followed by the number of standard 0.75 litre bottles each contains, according to whether it is champagne, Bordeaux or Burgundy.

The method

☆ As always, it is worth dividing the task up into bite-sized chunks. There are 14 names, so it would make sense to learn the names in threes, with an odd two at the end.

☆ Start by getting all the names off pat and in the right order. A mnemonic for each section might help. You could start with something like, 'Picking champagne for dinner?' I'll leave the rest up to you. You'll remember one you made yourself much better than a tailor-made one of mine.

☆ Learning the sizes is much harder – which is why we have produced an illustrated chart that you can learn to visualize in your mind's eye.

☆ It helps that the sizes are in ascending order which at least gives you a context in which to learn them.

☆ Finally, there are some bottles that simply don't exist (for example, there is no Picolo of anything except champagne). These are marked with a red dot on the table.

Now try these questions:

1 What do you call a bottle of champagne?
2 What is the smallest bottle of Bordeaux called?
3 What is the very largest bottle size?
4 How many normal bottles make a Methuselah?
5 What do 16 normal bottles make?
6 What size is a Magnum?
7 What is an Imperial?
8 How many bottles make a Rehoboam?
9 Can you have a Nebuchadnezzar of champagne?
10 What is a Filette?

NAME	CHAMPAGNE	BORDEAUX	BURGUNDY
Picolo	¼	•	•
Chopine	•	⅓	•
Filette/Demi	½	½	½
Magnum	2	2	2
Marie Jeanne	•	3	•
Double Magnum	•	4	•
Jeroboam	4	6	4
Rehoboam	6	•	6
Imperial	•	8	•
Methuselah	8	•	8
Salmanazar	12	•	12
Balthazar	16	16	16
Nebuchadnezzar	20	20	20
Melchior	24	24	24

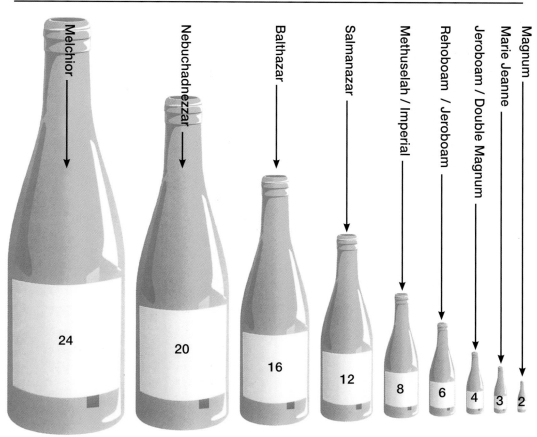

LONG-TERM MEMORY TASK

Learn the Beaufort Scale

TIME: **1 hour** LEVEL: **Hard**

The Beaufort Scale describes wind speed. It may not form part of your everyday conversation, but it has its uses, even for those of us who never go to sea and only concern ourselves with the weather when wondering whether or not to take a brolly when we go out.

Instructions

☆ The scale is always quoted in the form Force 1, Force 2, and so on, so start by learning each force with its brief description (such as Force 1, calm).

☆ When you have memorized these, you can add in the more detailed descriptions. Picture the scene to bring each force vividly to mind.

☆ Finally, you can add in the actual wind speeds. Only learn the speed in knots if you are really keen (or go sailing).

☆ Practise in real situations. Make a point of estimating the wind speed wherever you go (you should be able to check your estimates on a weather map afterwards).

☆ Use your real-life experiences to reinforce your memorization. After a while, you should be able to tell the force of the wind just by the way it feels and sounds, and the effect it has on the environment.

FORCE	EQUIVALENT SPEED *10 m (11 yds) above ground*		DESCRIPTION	EFFECTS
	miles/hour	knots		
0	0–1	0–1	Calm	Calm; smoke rises vertically.
1	1–3	1–3	Light air	Direction of wind shown by smoke drift, but not by wind vanes.
2	4–7	4–6	Light breeze	Wind felt on face; leaves rustle; ordinary vanes moved by wind.
3	8–12	7–10	Gentle breeze	Leaves and small twigs in constant motion; wind extends light flag.
4	13–18	11–16	Moderate breeze	Raises dust and loose paper; small branches are moved.
5	19–24	17–21	Fresh breeze	Small trees in leaf begin to sway; crested wavelets form on inland waters.
6	25–31	22–27	Strong breeze	Large branches in motion; whistling heard in telegraph wires; umbrellas used with difficulty.
7	32–38	28–33	Near gale	Whole trees in motion; inconvenience felt when walking against the wind.
8	39–46	34–40	Gale	Breaks twigs off trees; generally impedes progress.
9	47–54	41–47	Severe gale	Slight structural damage occurs (chimney-pots and slates removed).
10	55–63	48–55	Storm	Seldom experienced inland; trees uprooted; considerable structural damage occurrs.
11	64–72	56–63	Violent storm	Very rarely experienced; accompanied by widespread damage.
12	73–83	64–71	Hurricane	–

LONG-TERM MEMORY TASK

Roman numerals

TIME: **20 minutes** LEVEL: **Easy**

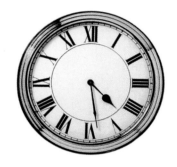

We all know some Roman numerals, but many of us get stuck on numbers larger than ten. Here is a complete list for you to learn. When you feel confident that you know the whole lot, you can try the test below.

Instructions

Roman numerals are very easy once you have the trick of them. Within each number, anything to the left of the largest numeral is subtracted from it, for example: IV is actually 5–1 = 4. CM is 1000–100 = 900. Anything to the right of the largest numeral is added to it, for example LV = 50 + 5 = 55. XV = 10 + 5 = 15. Once you have learned these basic principles, you only have to remember a few special letters – C, D, L and M. If you want to be able to work with huge numbers, you have to learn that a numeral with an overscore is multiplied by 1000. Thus V, which is normally 5, is 5000 if it is overscored. Isn't that simple?

1	**I**	30	**XXX**	600	**DC**
2	**II**	40	**XL**	700	**DCC**
3	**III**	50	**L**	800	**DCCC**
4	**IV**	60	**LX**	900	**CM**
5	**V**	70	**LXX**	1000	**M**
6	**VI**	80	**LXXX**	5000	**$\overline{V}$**
7	**VII**	90	**XC**	10000	**$\overline{X}$**
8	**VIII**	100	**C**	50000	**$\overline{L}$**
9	**IX**	200	**CC**	100000	**$\overline{C}$**
10	**X**	400	**CD**	500000	**$\overline{D}$**
20	**XX**	500	**D**	1000000	**$\overline{M}$**

Now try to convert these numbers into Roman numerals:

15	35	239
426	5244	7890
45859		

Check your answers on page 157.

VISUAL MEMORY TASK

Memorizing unusual capital cities

TIME: **1 hour** LEVEL: **Hard**

I once had a job with a firm that published atlases, and it was then that I discovered just how ignorant many people (including myself) are about geography. They might well know the capitals of places such as the US, France and Germany, but if you ask them to find anywhere a little more exotic, they fall down in a heap. This is therefore a useful exercise in that it will not only improve your powers of memory, but also increase your store of geographical knowledge. We have deliberately chosen 34 of the lesser-known capitals for you to memorize. Turn to pages 110–111 to view the map of the world.

Instructions

1 Learn one area of the world at a time.
2 Use the map to help you learn not only the countries and their capitals, but also where the countries are in relation to the rest of the world. The better your visual memory is, the easier you will find this task.

3 Don't make the mistake of merely learning the countries and capitals as lists of words. Putting them all in their *correct geographical context* will increase their value ten-fold.

4 Once you have learned these capitals you can extend your geographical knowledge. Why not add other countries and, as well as capitals, add other major cities, rivers, mountains, in fact anything that takes your fancy. You'll find that creating your own mental world map can be fun and is actually useful.

	Country	Capital City		Country	Capital City
1	Angola	Luanda	18	Indonesia	Jakarta
2	Bangladesh	Dhaka	19	Jamaica	Kingston
3	Barbados	Bridgetown	20	Laos	Vientiane
4	Burkina Faso	Ouagadougou	21	Liberia	Monrovia
5	Costa Rica	San Jose	22	Madagascar	Antananarivo
6	Dominica	Roseau	23	Mali	Bamako
7	Ecuador	Quito	24	Mongolia	Ulaanbaatar
8	Equatorial Guinea	Malabo	25	Mauritius	Port Louis
9	Eritrea	Asmara	26	Morocco	Rabat
10	Gabon	Libreville	27	Oman	Muscat
11	Gambia	Banjul	28	Paraguay	Asuncion
12	Georgia	Tbilisi	29	Qatar	Doha
13	Grenada	St George's	30	Seychelles	Victoria
14	Guinea	Conakry	31	Somalia	Mogadishu
15	Guyana	Georgetown	32	Surinam	Paramaribo
16	Haiti	Port-au-Prince	33	Taiwan	Taipei
17	Honduras	Tegucigalpa	34	Uzbekistan	Tashkent

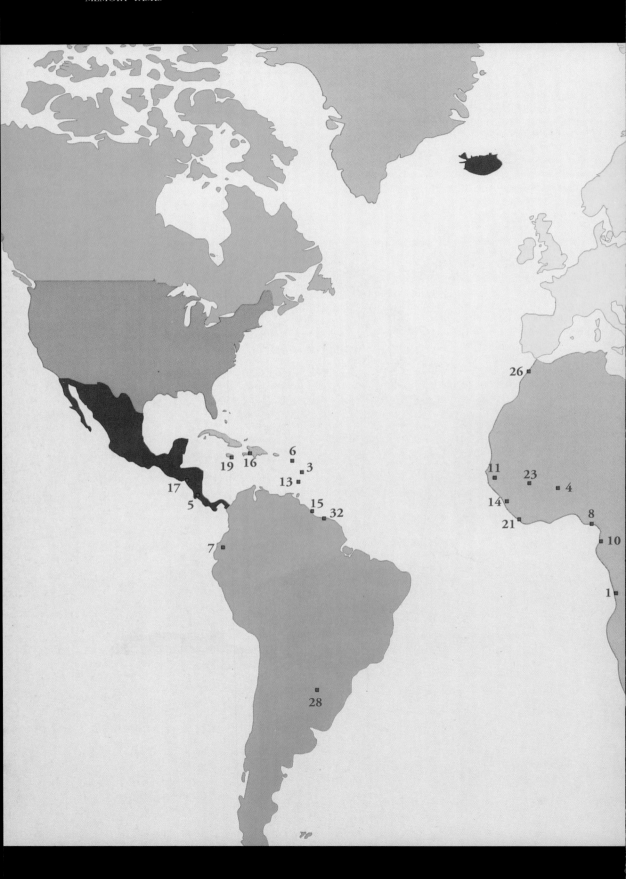

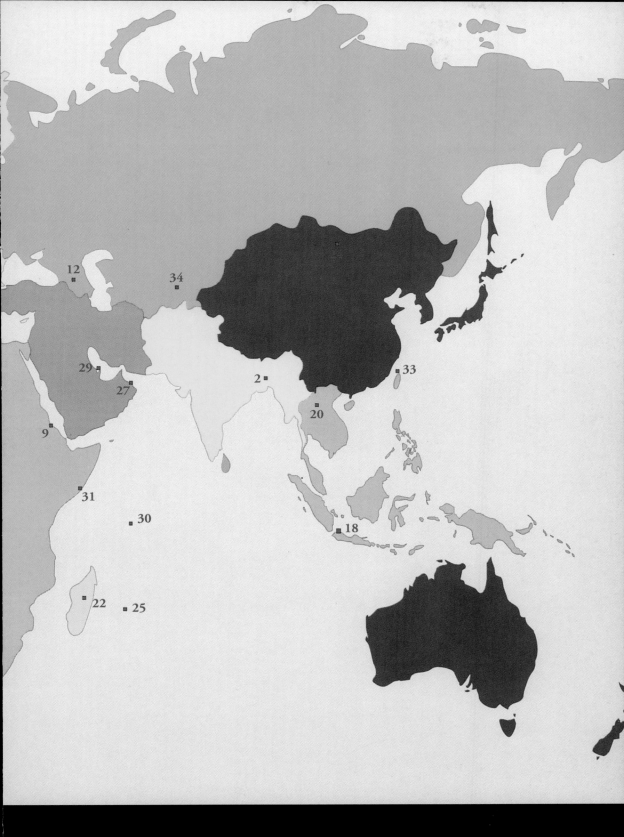

VISUAL MEMORY TASK

Memorizing cloud types

TIME: **20 minutes** LEVEL: **Medium**

The attraction of this exercise is that it is not only of some practical use (because it helps you to predict the weather with some accuracy), but it also involves using several types of memory. What's more, you can practise this exercise every day and as often as you want by doing no more than looking out of the window.

Instructions

☆ First, learn what the basic words mean:

Cumulus	=	heap
Stratus	=	layer
Cirrus	=	curl
Nimbus	=	rain

☆ Once you have the meanings in mind, it is much easier to relate the words to the pictures.

☆ Remember that the altitudes work from the highest to the lowest and go in bands (for example, the first three are all exactly the same, which makes them easy to remember).

☆ Use the picture and say the name as you touch each cloud type.

☆ Once you know them in the highest-to-lowest order, try to learn them out of order as well.

☆ Practise on real clouds whenever you go out.

REF	CLOUD NAME	CLOUD HEIGHT	DESCRIPTION
High clouds			
A	Cirrus	*5000–13700m*	High, detached, white filaments of wispy cloud.
B	Cirrocumulus	*5000–13700m*	'Mackerel sky' – grains or ripples of white cloud in regular patterns.
C	Cirrostratus	*5000–13700m*	Sheets of cloud covering large areas of the sky, sometimes producing a halo effect.
Middle clouds			
D	Altocumulus	*2000–7000m*	Patches and sheets of rounded clouds separate or merged.
E	Altostratus	*2000–7000m*	Sheets of grey-blue cloud, often obscuring sun and moon.

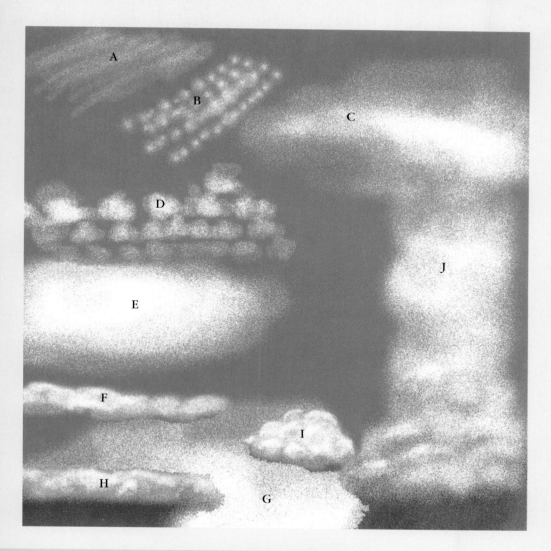

REF	CLOUD NAME	CLOUD HEIGHT	DESCRIPTION

Low clouds

REF	CLOUD NAME	CLOUD HEIGHT	DESCRIPTION
F	**Stratocumulus**	*460–2000m*	Layers of white cloud with grey areas; often bringing light rain or snow.
G	**Stratus**	*Surface–460m*	Uniform low grey cloud; outline of sun and moon visible where cloud is thin.
H	**Nimbostratus**	*900–3000m*	Associated with rain and snow, often covering most of the sky – dark and heavy.

Clouds of vertical development

REF	CLOUD NAME	CLOUD HEIGHT	DESCRIPTION
I	**Cumulus**	*460–2000m*	Heaped, cauliflower shape; brilliant white with dark base.
J	**Cumulonimbus**	*460–2000m*	Heavy, dense cloud with huge towers and shadows at base.

PROCEDURAL MEMORY TASK
Learn semaphore

TIME: **1 hour** LEVEL: **Hard**

The chances of semaphore being of practical use to you are, I admit, slight. However, that is not the point. This exercise is a wonderful example of learning by doing. It gives you a chance to combine the intellectual process of learning with the use of what might be called body memory. Your body is excellent at remembering things, so good, in fact, that much of the time you are quite unaware of what it is doing. Take riding a bike, for example. Once you have the knack of it, you never have to think about balance again, because your muscles remember how it's done. You only have to consciously take over at moments when things go badly wrong and a major correction is called for.

Of course, strictly speaking, the muscles are not themselves repositories of memory. But you do become very good at interpreting messages from your body and responding to them automatically. Learning semaphore will give you a chance to hone that skill a little further. Note that the figures in the diagrams opposite are facing you.

Instructions

1 Start by going through the letters in strict alphabetical order, saying the name of each letter out loud as you make the appropriate signal.

2 As always, break your task into chunks. Learn only a few letters at a time and, once you are sure of them, learn a few more.

3 Perfect your skill by reproducing the letters in a random order. If possible, get someone to hold the book and call out letters at random to which you must respond with the right signals.

4 Bear in mind that, as with all coded signals, context gives you some good clues. With practice, you won't have to stumble along, painstakingly translating one word at a time, but will be able to predict what comes next.

5 Experienced signallers use abbreviated forms, much like people sending text messages on their mobile phones. So, if you ever have to use semaphore for real, make sure you abbreviate.

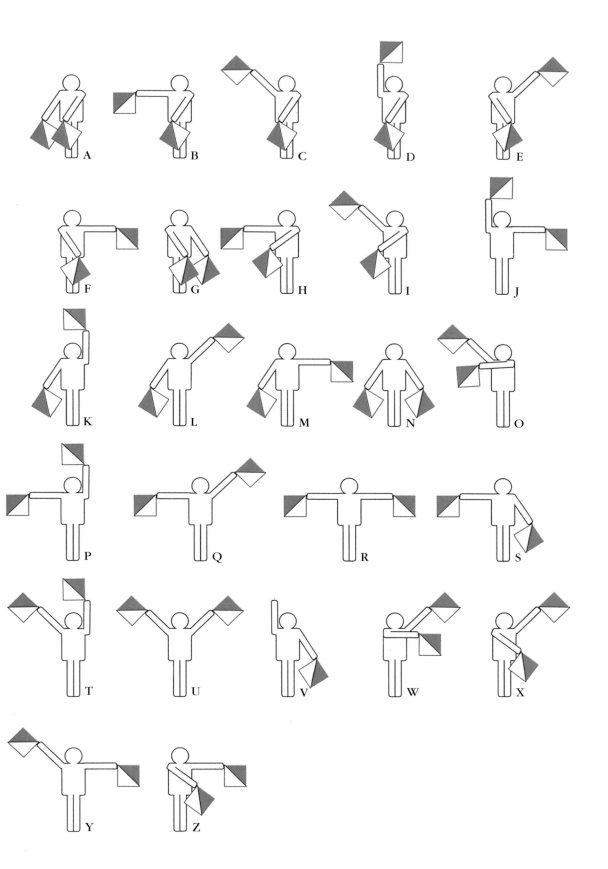

Test yourself by translating the follow semaphore messages:

1

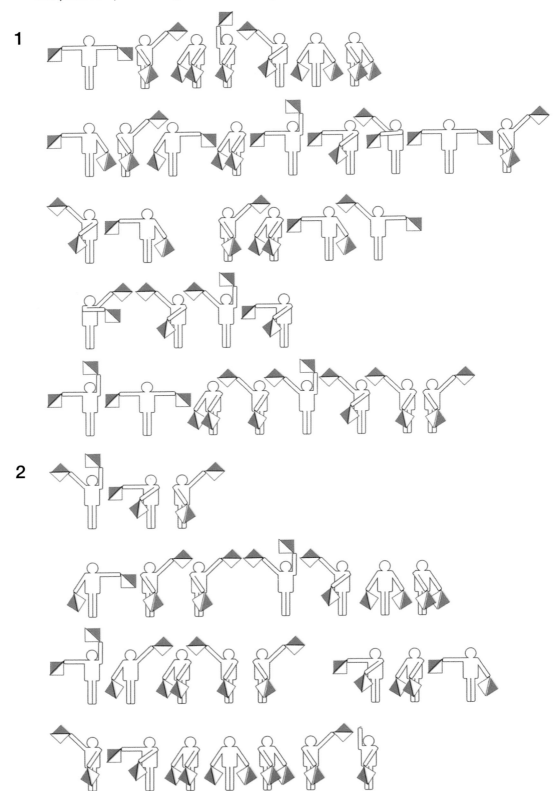

2

3

4

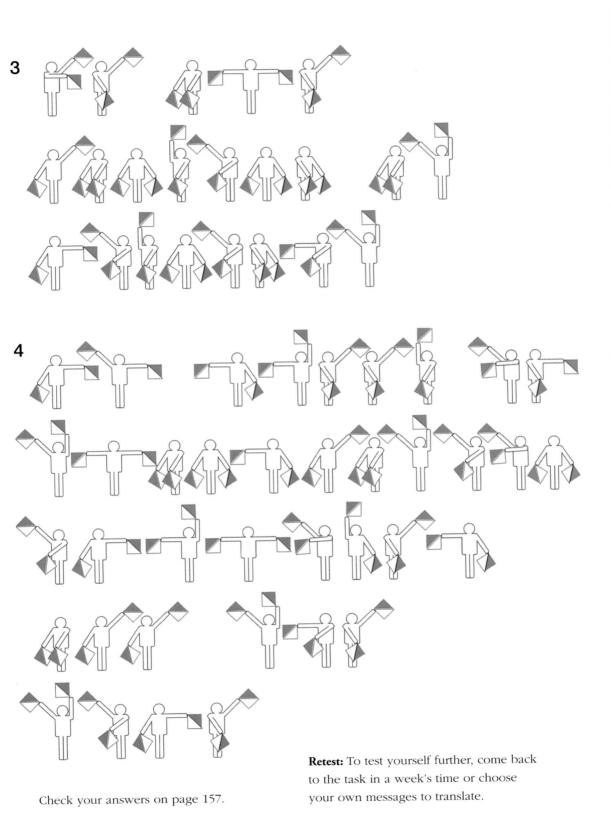

Check your answers on page 157.

Retest: To test yourself further, come back to the task in a week's time or choose your own messages to translate.

VISUAL MEMORY TASK
Learn Morse code

TIME: **30 minutes** LEVEL: **Easy**

You may think that you'll never need to know Morse code, but it is easy to learn and can be surprisingly useful. Younger readers might like to use it as a 'secret' code. It is a great way of sharpening your 'doing' memory skills (see page 13).

Instructions

1 First, look at the code and work through it from A–Z (plus 0–9 and the punctuation marks).
2 As you go through, say it out loud (traditionally you say 'dah' for a dash and 'dit' for a dot).
3 As you say the code, also tap it out with a pencil on your desk or table. A heavy tap represents a dash and a light one is a dot.
4 Once you can do the whole alphabet in the correct order, you have to be able to do it out of order. Get a friend to test you.
5 You have finished this task when you can produce any letter, numeral or punctuation mark on request.

Tap out the following messages from memory

☆ This is your captain speaking.

☆ The ship is listing hard to starboard.

☆ We appear to be sinking fast.

☆ Do you want us to man the lifeboats?

☆ Land has been sighted on the port side.

☆ How much food and water remain?

☆ Report your position. How many survivors are there?

☆ We will send our medical officer to care for your wounded.

☆ When we reach port there will have to be an enquiry.

☆ There is a report of an explosion aboard your ship.

If you have become hooked on Morse you need to work at increasing your speed, and there are Morse code websites that will help you do this.

Here is the code

A	.-	U	..-
B	-...	V	...-
C	-.-.	W	.--
D	-..	X	-..-
E	.	Y	-.--
F	..-.	Z	--..
G	--.	0	-----
H	....	1	.----
I	..	2	..---
J	.---	3	...--
K	-.-	4	....-
L	.-..	5	.....
M	--	6	-....
N	-.	7	--...
O	---	8	---..
P	.--.	9	----.
Q	--.-		
R	.-.	Full stop	.-.-.-
S	...	Comma	--..--
T	-	Query	..--..

VISUAL MEMORY TASK

Memorize something really confusing

TIME: **30 minutes** LEVEL: **Hard**

The table below is a particular form of mental torment introduced to me by my daughter, Gina. It contains the names of a number of colours and things associated with colours. However, they have been coloured incorrectly – except for a few which, to make things more confusing, are in the correct colours. Trying to memorize this information is difficult simply because there is a voice at the back of your mind constantly saying, 'This does not compute!' The trick is to be able to learn what is actually in front of you, rather than what you think should be there.

RED	SILVER	LEMON
HOLLY	YELLOW	GREEN
BLUE	BLACK	WHITE
GRASS	VIOLET	BROWN
EMERALD	IVY	BANANA
GOLD	COAL	SEA
BROWN	MILK	SUN
ORANGE	SAND	APPLE
BUTTER	GREY	INDIGO
PURPLE	SKY	TAN

Instructions

1 The way to learn all this is to start with the words and forget for a moment about the colours. Simply learn the words in columns from left to right. Number the columns 1–3 and the rows 1–10.

2 If you want, you can create a mnemonic from the initial letters in each column.

3 Now, close your eyes and start to visualize the colours. Try to see a picture of each column in your mind's eye. If it helps, you can say to yourself, RED is green, GREEN is black, VIOLET is blue, or you can create a mnemonic for the initial letters of the colours as well.

4 Whichever way you do it, this is a tough test. When you think you have the whole table memorized, cover the page and try the questions, right. They start out simple but get much tougher as they go along.

Colour test

1 What colour is BUTTER?

2 What colour is BANANA?

3 Which column (numbering from the left) is SEA in?

4 What is to the left of COAL and what colour is it?

5 What comes below APPLE?

6 What is to the right of GREY?

7 What colour is the word between TAN and PURPLE?

8 What is two places below YELLOW?

9 What is one place above, and one place to the right, of VIOLET?

10 How many words are in the correct colours?

11 Name all the words printed on green.

12 Name the five words printed on black.

13 Which is the lower of the two words printed in bright blue?

14 What are the two bright blue words and where are they?

15 Which word printed in dark blue do you associate with green?

Comprehension
TIME: **10 minutes** LEVEL: **Medium**

You might have had to do something like this when you were at school. But this one is a real toughie. What follows is a short passage containing quite a lot of detail. Your task is to read it thoroughly once and then answer the questions.

Instructions

There is no easy way to learn all this. Read the piece slowly and carefully. Go over each sentence a number of times and make sure you understand it. One way to fix everything in your memory would be to list all the characters and write down what you know about each. You could also draw arrows to show who is emotionally linked to whom. If you can't get more than a few questions right, go back to the beginning and give yourself another chance.

Every Friday night, Jeff meets up with his friends, Pete, Laura, Sue, Graham, Mark, Sinead and Sophie. Sometimes they go out for dinner and they prefer Italian, though Laura can't eat pasta and Mark dislikes pepperoni. Occasionally they go for a curry, and their favourite place is the Maharajah just near the cinema in the Market Place. They used to go to the Taj Mahal but stopped because Graham found some undercooked chicken in his vindaloo. Pete and Laura got engaged last Christmas. Jeff used to go out with Laura but they split up a year ago. He'd like to go out with Sinead but she only has eyes for Mark. Sue had a bit of a thing with Graham for a while but now they've split up and she keeps talking about moving back to Wales to be near her elderly parents. Laura and Sue are lawyers and Sophie works in a bank. Sinead is a photographer and is in partnership with Jeff.

Now answer these questions:
1. Who did Sue go out with for a while?
2. Who are the photographers?
3. Who doesn't like pepperoni?
4. Why did they stop eating at the Taj Mahal?
5. Which is their favourite Indian restaurant?
6. Who can't eat pasta?
7. Which of the characters is Welsh?
8. Who are the lawyers?
9. Where does Sophie work?
10. Which building is near the Maharajah restaurant?
11. Which night do the friends usually meet up?
12. Who did Jeff go out with?
13. Which part of town is the cinema in?
14. When did Pete and Laura get engaged?
15. Who is Sinead in love with?

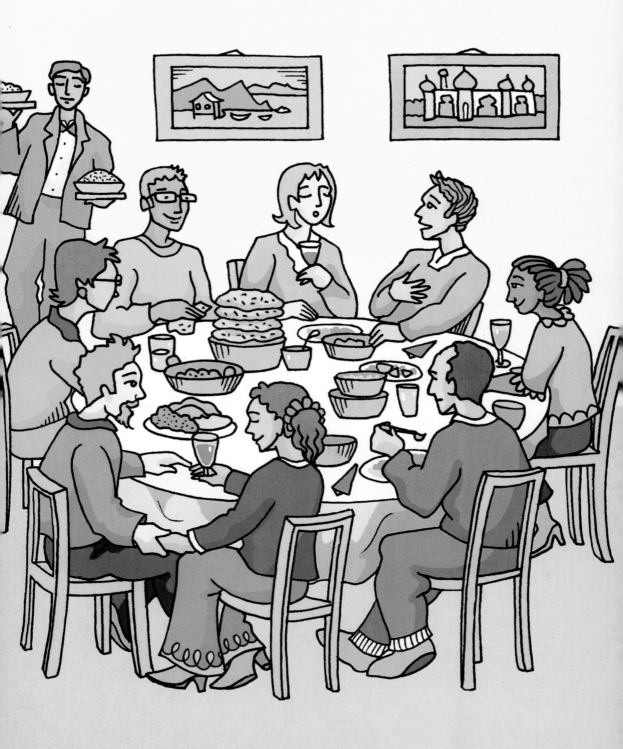

Memorize a table of symbols

TIME: **20 minutes** LEVEL: **Hard**

What makes this exercise so tough is that many of the symbols are unfamiliar. Some of them you won't even know by name. Obviously, it is much harder to memorize information that does not make much sense to us. But it can be done.

Instructions

1 Give names to all the symbols you don't know. Make up something that you find memorable (the sillier the better).

2 Make sure that you can remember all the names you have made up.

3 Spend some time memorizing the grid, first in columns from left to right, and then in rows from top to bottom.

4 Do one column or row at a time and make sure your memorization of that portion is perfect before you go on to the next.

5 If it helps, you can make up a mnemonic for each column and row using the initial letters of the symbols' names.

6 Try to record a picture of the grid in your mind's eye. Close your eyes and see the grid in front of you. This will take quite a lot of concentration.

7 Now, produce a set of blank grids (this is easily done on a computer) and try filling in the information you remember. Keep checking back with the diagram and correcting mistakes.

When you feel confident that you know the whole grid by heart, try the test below:

1 Which symbol is at the top of the fourth column from the left?
2 Which symbol is to the right of ≈ ?
3 What comes directly below ?
4 Where in which row (numbering from the top) is the ✓
5 Which symbol is to the left of * ?
6 Write down or draw all the symbols in the middle column.
7 Draw all the symbols on the bottom row.
8 Is ◊ in a higher or lower row than ≠ ?
9 What is at the end of the row that starts with ❋ ?
10 What is diagonally below ∞ ?
11 Where is π?
12 What is at the bottom of the column that has ✪ at the top?
13 What is three places to the right of ❐ ?
14 What comes three places above * ?
15 What comes at the end of the row that starts with ± ?

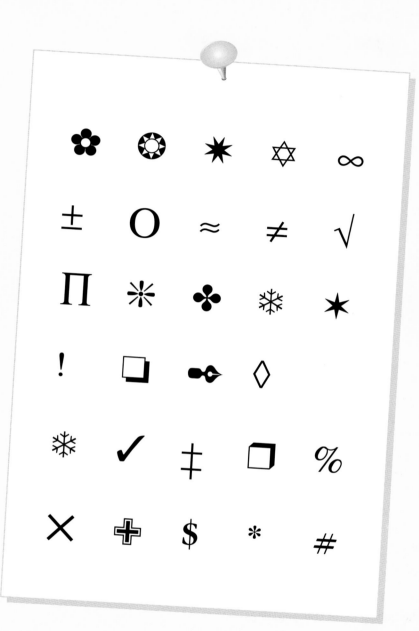

PROCEDURAL MEMORY

Learning to tie knots

TIME: **20 minutes** LEVEL: **Medium**

This is the ultimate exercise for those who wish to develop their 'doing' memory (see page 13). Tying knots can be a very complicated business and describing the process in words often makes things worse rather than better. Thus this becomes entirely a visual/kinaesthetic exercise in which words play no part. I have chosen some knots that are complicated enough to present a challenge, but simple enough not to require any previous experience.

Instructions

The only way to remember how to tie a knot is with your fingertips. Visual cues will, of course, also play a part but you will mostly just have to feel your way to success. Elsewhere in the book I have pointed out that mere repetition is not a very strong memory glue. The skill of knot-tying is an exception. You will need to practise each knot many times before you get it exactly right.

Retest: Reviewing your knot-tying skills is particularly important if you want to keep them current. This sort of memory evaporates rapidly if not practised regularly.

The knots
Blood bight

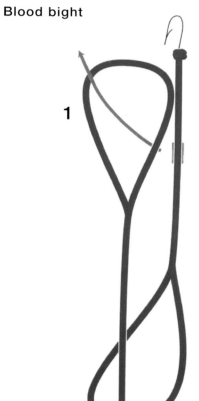

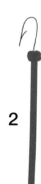

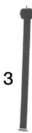

True lover's knot

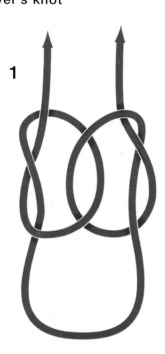

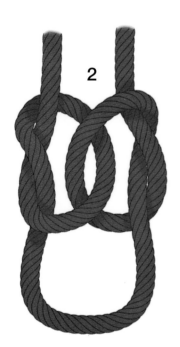

Surgeon's knot

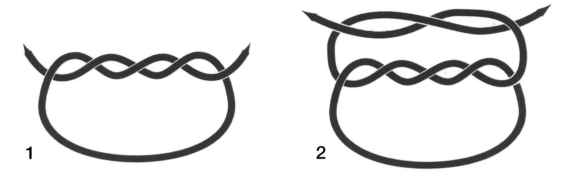

Shamrock knot

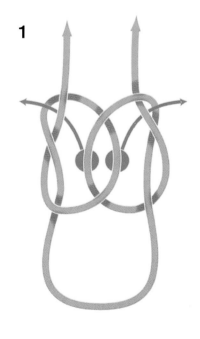

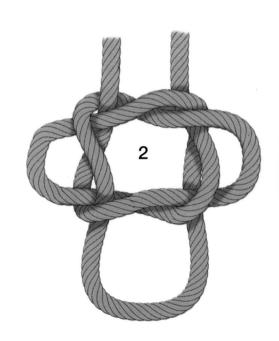

Jug sling

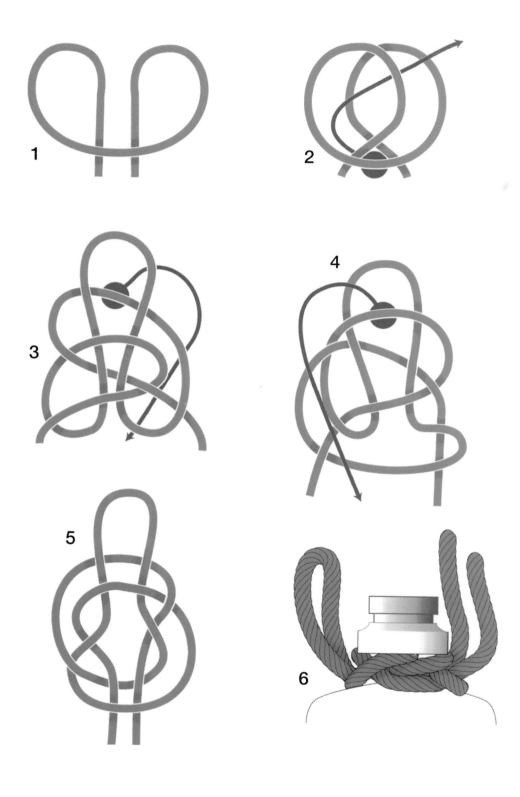

Learning long words
TIME: **20 minutes** LEVEL: **Hard**

If you were a certain type of kid at school you might have whiled away some time learning how to spell 'antidisestablishmentarianism' and other similarly interesting but useless words. In this exercise you will memorize a number of words that are equally fascinating and, let's face it, equally useless. So why bother? Just because learning this sort of complex information is a good way of building up brain muscle.

Rehearsing long words in quiet moments (on boring journeys, for example) is an easy way to keep your new memory skills in good shape.

Instructions
Long words are absolutely ideal for the 'divide and conquer' method. Most of them look fearsome when spelled out in full, but are actually made up of familiar components or, at least, are composed of sounds that are easy to remember.

☆ I have split the words below not into syllables but into chunks that I find easy to remember. Should you find that the splits I have chosen do not suit you, feel free to choose your own. It may help to write the words down as you spell them.

☆ Always spell out loud because the listening process is an important way to help you learn.

☆ Some people like to write words with a fingertip in the palm of their hand. This stimulates their touch memory.

Honorificabilitudinity
Honor / ifi / cabili / tudi / nity
I have made three of the chunks end in 'i' to make them more memorable.
Meaning = the quality of being honorable.

Dihydroxylphenylalanine
Di / hydroxyl / pheny / lala / nine
Remember to pronounce the first chunk to rhyme with 'dye' or you might introduce an 'e' by mistake. Those with scientific training might like to keep the third chunk as phenyl because this makes sense to scientists, but I divided it the way I did because I thought that, for most people, 'lala' would be more memorable than 'ala'.
Meaning = dopamine, an animo acid.

Gynotikolobomassophile
Gyno / tiko / lobo /masso /phile
Once you've made all but the last chunk end in an 'o', this one becomes a piece of cake.
Meaning = someone who likes to nibble women's earlobes.

Hexamethylenetetramine

Hexa / methyl / ene / tetra / mine

This is probably easier if you pronounce 'ene' to rhyme with 'meany' rather than any. *Meaning = a specific organic compound.*

Bathysiderodromophobia

Bathy / side / rod / romo / phobia

Again, if you understand the elements of this word you might wish to split it differently (using 'sidero' and 'dromo', for example). My split is for those to whom the word is just a meaningless jumble. *Meaning = an irrational fear of being underground.*

Rhombicosidodecahedron

Rhombi / cosi / dodeca / hedron

The silent 'h' in 'rhombi' might escape you unless you make a point of pronouncing it to yourself. *Meaning = a specific 62-faced geometric solid.*

Pseudomonocotyledonous

Pseudo / mono / coty / ledo / nous

This one is really easy, even though it is longer than any you have tried so far. Give thanks, and add quickly to your store of knowledge. *Meaning = having two coalescent cotyledons.*

Hippopotomonstrosesquippedaliophobia

Hippo / poto / monstro / sesquip / pedalio / phobia

Again, I have made as many of the chunks as possible end in 'o'. 'Hippo', 'monstro' and 'phobia' are all elements that should be familiar to you. *Meaning = fear of long words.*

Hepaticocholangiocholecystenterostomies

Hepati / cocho / langi / ocho / lecy / stent / eros / tomies

Once you can remember how to say this one (which should only take you a couple of minutes) the spelling is a piece of cake.
Meaning = a surgical connection between the gall bladder and the hepatic duct.

Pneumonoultramicroscopicsilicovolcanoconiosis

Pneumono / ultra / micro / scopic / sili / covol / cano / coni / osis

This one is often quoted in lists of long words. *Meaning = a rather nasty lung disease.*

Aequeosalinocalcalinosetaceoaluminosocupreovitriolic

Aequeo / salino / calcalino / seta / ceo / alumino / socu / preo / vitriolic
Meaning = a description of the spa waters at Bath, England.

Osseocarnisanguineoviscericartilagninonervomedullary

Osseo / carni / sanguin / eo / visceri / cartil / agnino / nervo / medullary
Meaning = a lung disease.

LONG-TERM MEMORY TASK

Learn the battles of the American Civil War

TIME: **1 hour** LEVEL: **Hard**

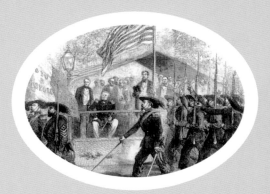

This task is a perfect example of the way in which understanding helps memory. It is perfectly possible to learn this list of battles by the old-fashioned rote method. If, however, you take the trouble to learn the story of the war (even if only in outline), the events start to make more sense and become more memorable. For a proper understanding, you should go to a website such as: http://www.historyplace.com for a complete explanation of who did what to whom and why.

Instructions

I have split up the war into years, so that you can learn it a bit at a time (the source I took the information from presented it in one large slab, which made it almost completely indigestible).

☆ You might like to create a mnemonic for each year of the war using the initials of battle names.

☆ The years are quite easy to remember because there are few of them, but you will have difficulty with the months and days. Practise writing out your own list for each year. Keep writing it over and over again and read what you are writing out loud to yourself.

☆ Read an abbreviated account of the war and make your own summary, so that you can put your information in context. The more you understand the context, the easier it will be to remember the details.

☆ Get someone to test you by asking for battle names and dates at random.

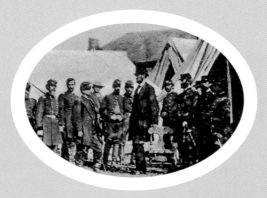

BATTLE	DATE	SITE
1861		
1st Battle of Bull Run	21 July 1861	Manasses, Virginia
1862		
Fort Henry	6 February 1862	W. Tennessee
Fort Donelson	16 February 1862	W. Tennessee
Shiloh	6–7 April 1862	Pittsburgh Landing, W. Tennessee
Battle of Seven Days	25 June–1 July 1862	Virginia
2nd Battle of Bull Run	27–30 August 1862	Manassas, Virginia
Antietam	17 September 1862	Antietam Creek, Marylan
Fredericksburg	13 December 1862	Fredericksburg, Virginia
1863		
Chancellorship	1–4 May 1863	Chancellorship, Virginia
Siege of Vicksburg	19 May–4 July 1863	Vicksburg, Virginia
Gettysburg	1–3 July 1863	Gettysburg, Pennsylvania
Chickamauga	19–20 September 1863	Chickamauga, Georgia
Chattanooga	23–25 November 1863	Chattanooga, Tennessee
1864		
Battle of the Wilderness	5–9 May 1864	Northern Virginia
Spotsylvania	May 1864	Spotsylvania, Virginia
Cold Harbor	3 June 1864	Virginia
Siege of Petersburg	20 June 1864–2 April 1865	Petersburg, Virginia
Mobile Bay	5 August 1864	Alabama
Atlanta	2 September 1864	Georgia
Nashville	15–16 December 1864	Tennessee
1865 (Surrenders)		
Lee surrenders to Grant	9 April 1865	Appomattox, Virginia
Johnson surrenders to Sherman	17 April 1865	Raleigh, North Carolina

LONG-TERM MEMORY TASK
The Periodic Table of the elements

TIME: **2 hours** LEVEL: **Hard**

You will probably take one look at the Periodic Table and think, 'No way am I learning that!' But wait just a moment. It really isn't as hard as you might think and though even scientists mostly rely on a physical chart hanging on the laboratory wall, there is no reason why you shouldn't commit the whole thing to memory.

Instructions

☆ First, note that the whole structure bears some resemblance to a fort (OK, you have to use a little imagination

here). But it is built out of blocks and has numbers across the top and side. Therefore, the first thing you need to do is master this structure.

☆ For the moment, practise drawing just the block without any reference to the symbols for the elements. Remember how many blocks go in each column and where the blanks are. Keep the picture of the whole structure in your mind's eye as you draw.

	1	2	3	4	5	6	7	8	9
1	H 1 Hydrogen								
2	Li 3 Lithium	Be 4 Beryllium							
3	Na 11 Sodium	Mg 12 Magnesium							
4	K 19 Potassium	Ca 20 Calcium	Sc 21 Scandium	Ti 22 Titanium	V 23 Vanadium	Cr 24 Chromium	Mn 25 Manganese	Fe 26 Iron	Co 27 Cobalt
5	Rb 37 Rubidium	Sr 38 Strontium	Y 39 Yttrium	Zr 40 Zirconium	Nb 41 Niobium	Mo 42 Molybdenum	Tc 43 Technetium	Ru 44 Ruthenium	Rh 45 Rhodium
6	Cs 55 Caesium	Ba 56* Barium	Lu 71 Lutetium	Hf 72 Hafnium	Ta 73 Tantalum	W 74 Tungsten	Re 75 Rhenium	Os 76 Osmium	Ir 77 Iridium
7	Fr 87 Francium	Ra 88** Radium	Lr 103 Lawrencium	Rf 104 Rutherfordium	Db 105 Dubnium	Sg 106 Seaborgium	Bh 107 Bohrium	Hs 108 Hassium	Mt 109 Meitnerium
* Lanthanoids		La 57 Lanthanum	Ce 58 Cerium	Pr 59 Praseodymium	Nd 60 Neodymium	Pm 61 Promethium	Sm 62 Samarium	Eu 63 Europium
** Actinoids		Ac 89 Actinium	Th 90 Thorium	Pa 91 Protactinium	U 92 Uranium	Np 93 Neptunium	Pu 94 Plutonium	Am 95 Americium

☆ Now learn the elements and their symbols. The good news is that many of the names are part of our normal vocabulary.

☆ The next bit of good news is that almost all of the symbols are merely contractions of the full names. So, though you might not be familiar with cobalt, you won't struggle with the notion that its symbol is Co. All you then have to do is struggle with the exceptions. If you did chemistry at school, even for a few years, you will probably remember some of the exceptions, such as Fe for Iron and Cu for Copper.

☆ Use the numbered columns to help split the table into learnable chunks.

☆ We have included the symbols with their full names beside them. Note that a lot of the columns have only four names in them.

☆ Finally, learn the Lanthanoids and Actinoids. As you can see, they form a block under the main table, so you can either learn them as an add-on to each column or think of them as a separate entity.

10	11	12	13	14	15	16	17	18
								He 2 Helium
			B 5 Boron	C 6 Carbon	N 7 Nitrogen	O 8 Oxygen	F 9 Fluorine	Ne 10 Neon
			Al 13 Aluminum	Si 14 Silicon	P 15 Phosphorus	S 16 Sulphur	Cl 17 Chlorine	Ar 18 Argon
Ni 28 Nickel	Cu 29 Copper	Zn 30 Zinc	Ga 31 Gallium	Ge 32 Germanium	As 33 Arsenic	Se 34 Selenium	Br 35 Bromine	Kr 36 Krypton
Pd 46 Palladium	Ag 47 Silver	Cd 48 Cadmium	In 49 Indium	Sn 50 Tin	Sb 51 Antimony	Te 52 Tellurium	I 53 Iodine	Xe 54 Xenon
Pt 78 Platinum	Au 79 Gold	Hg 80 Mercury	Tl 81 Thallium	Tb 82 Lead	Bi 83 Bismuth	Po 84 Polonium	At 85 Astatine	Rn 86 Radon
Ds 110 Darmstadium	Uuu 111 Unununium	Uub 112 Ununbium	Uut 113 Ununtrium	Uuq 114 Ununquadium	Uup 115 Ununpentium	Uuh 116 Ununhexium	Uus 117 Ununseptium	Uud 118 Ununoctium
Gd 64 Gadolinium	Tb 65 Terbium	Dy 66 Dysprosium	Ho 67 Holmium	Er 68 Erbium	Tm 69 Thulium	Yb 70 Ytterbium		
Cm 96 Curium	Bk 97 Berkelium	Cf 98 Californium	Es 99 Einsteinium	Fm 100 Fermium	Md 101 Mendelevium	No 102 Nobelium		

VISUAL MEMORY TASK
Learn some basic Chinese characters
TIME: **10 minutes** LEVEL: **Easy**

This may look hard at first sight, but it is actually much simpler than you might think. Westerners seldom give any thought to Chinese writing, or assume that it is made up of random squiggles that must be a nightmare to learn. Not so. Chinese is very logical and has a number of basic building blocks, called radicals, that are not at all hard to learn. Many of the characters are actually simplified pictures, and this helps in remembering them.

Instructions

Look at the characters together with their translations. You'll find that the explanation written below each character will help fix it in your mind with ease. Within half an hour, you should have a fluent knowledge of twenty basic Chinese characters.

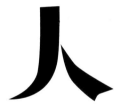 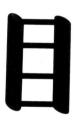

MAN
Looks like a pair of legs.

EAR
Looks a lot like an ear.

EYE
Looks a lot like a stylized picture of an eye.

FACE
Remember it as a portrait hanging on the wall.

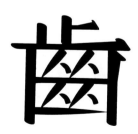 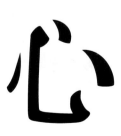 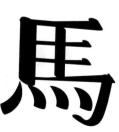 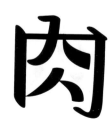

TEETH
This one requires a bit of imagination but you can see the teeth, can't you?

HEART
The three dots represent heartbeats.

HORSE
You can see four legs, the tail and the mane.

MEAT
Looks like a side of meat hanging in a butcher's shop.

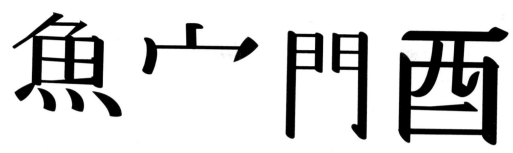

FISH
Head, scales and tail
are all visible.

ROOF
Quite obvious.
See the chimney?

GATE
Think of the saloon
doors in
an American Western.

JAR
Looks like a jar
with a stopper

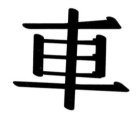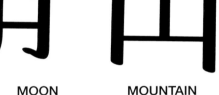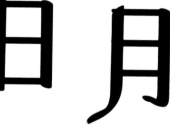

CART
This is the cart seen
from above. The
lines top and
bottom can then be
seen as wheels.

SUN
You'll see this in the
name for Japan,
which uses this
Chinese character
to describe itself as
the Land of the
Rising Sun.

MOON
Also means
'month', and you'll
see it on the
calendar that hangs
in your local
Chinese takeaway.

MOUNTAIN
You can see
three peaks.

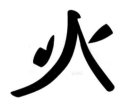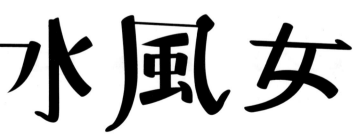

FIRE
Notice the rising
flames. If you see
'fire' and
'mountain' together
it means 'volcano'.

WATER
Not so obvious, but
a very important
and commonly seen
character.

WIND
A boat with sails
billowing in the
breeze. 'Wind' and
'water' together
means 'feng shui'.

WOMAN
A kneeling figure.

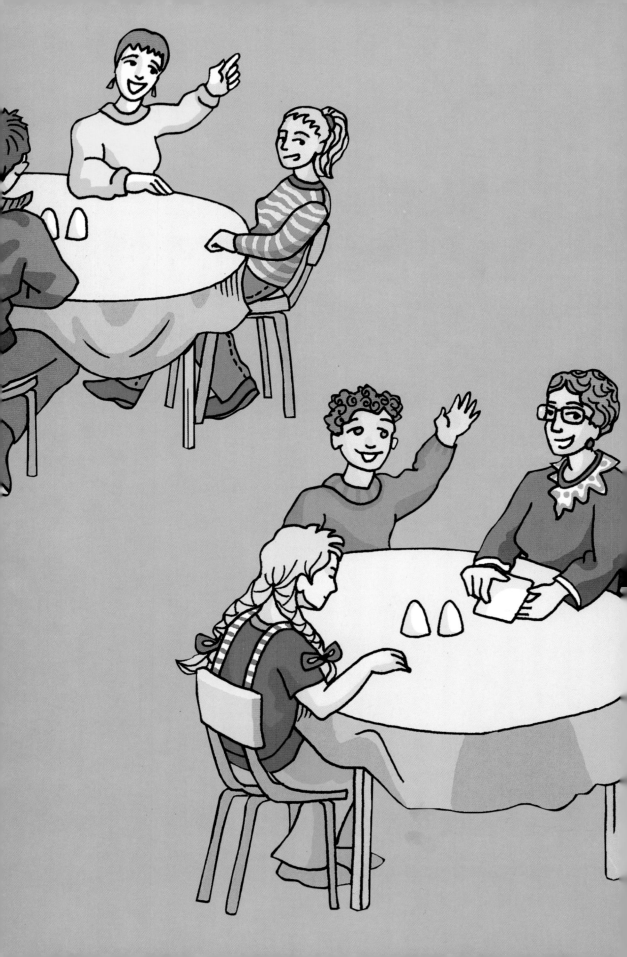

The Mammoth Memory Test

This is the place where you get to put your brand new, super-powered memory to the test. I realize that not all readers will have wanted to memorize everything in the Memory Tasks section, so what I have done is to split the test up so that you need only answer questions on subjects you feel comfortable with. That way you will end up with a score that says, 'Questions Attempted / Correct Answers'. You aren't expected to do the test without revision, so there is review time built into each section, but bear in mind that you have memorized the material before, so all you should need to bring it into sharp focus is a quick run-through. Even so, there is no point in trying to be a hero and then being disappointed because you haven't remembered as much as you thought you could. Attempt a section only when you are confident that you can get a good score.

The basic rules are, as ever:

- Divide and conquer (split tasks into chunks).

- Attack on all fronts (use as many methods as you can simultaneously).

- You don't have to do the whole test at one sitting.

... put your new super-powered memory to the test

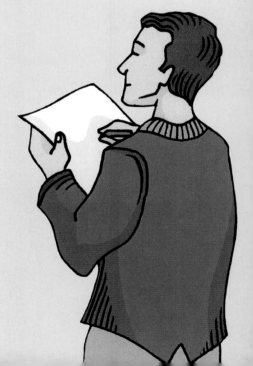

REVISION TASK 1

The alphabet backwards

(Pages 72–73)

Suggested revision: Write the alphabet out backwards once and sing it as you do so.

The test

Cover up your written effort. Go and do something else for a little while. Now see if you can sing the alphabet backwards.

A perfect performance	**5 points**
Anything less	**0 points**

REVISION TASK 2

The NATO phonetic alphabet

(Pages 74–75)

Suggested revision: Spend ten minutes revising the phonetic alphabet from the table.

The test

Read out the following in the phonetic alphabet. Try to read without pausing for thought. Pretend you're a cop reading out licence plates over the radio.

A 8 K 9 3 G 4

M 6 Z B 2 9 0

H D 4 3 J S T

U C W 6 Y N 8

D 5 E L P 5 3

F 6 J 1 2 K

Q 4 R V 9 X

For each line you get completely correct (without pausing): **10 points** Deduct **2 points** for each mistake and **1 point** if you had to pause.

Your score:

Your score:

REVISION TASK 3

Awkward spellings

(Pages 76–79)

Suggested revision: Go through the list and remind yourself of all the words you find hard to remember.

The test

Get someone to test you on fifteen words from your list at random.

Each correct spelling   **5 points**

REVISION TASK 4

Playing cards

(pages 80–81)

Suggested revision: Study the table again and see if you still have a picture of it stored in your mind's eye. If your original memorization was quirky enough it should still be with you (remember J-Lo as the Queen of Hearts?). Give yourself a few minutes to get it all into sharp focus again and then try these questions.

The test

1 Where is the 9 of Hearts?
2 Where is the Jack of Spades?
3 What comes above the Jack of Clubs?
4 Which card comes above the of Hearts?
5 What comes two places below the 10 of Clubs?
6 What is at the top of the middle column?
7 What is in the bottom right-hand corner?
8 What is in the very centre of the cards?
9 What comes at the end of the row that starts with the Jack of Hearts?
10 What is in the middle of the column that has the Queen of Diamonds at its bottom?

Each correct answer   **5 points**

Your score:

Your score:

REVISION TASK 5

I'm sorry I've forgotten your name

(Pages 82–83)

Suggested revision: Briefly look back at the pages and then answer the following questions.

The test

1 What is the name of the person wearing glasses?
2 What colour is Kelly's hair?
3 Does Miles Hill have a moustache?
4 What is Miss Lloyd's first name?
5 Who has red hair?
6 What is Tom's surname?
7 Whose nickname is 'Cornflake'?
8 What colour are Miss Dear's eyes and what is her first name?
9 How do you remember Carmen's name?
10 Who is 'Beaky'?
11 Recall Allen Levi's appearance.

Each correct answer   **5 points**

To build up your skills in this area, here is another set of names and faces to remember. Imagine you're at a party and have been introduced to various guests. Look at their names and faces for three minutes and try to fix them in your mind using the skills learned earlier in the book. Then cover the pictures. First, try to recall the faces in your mind's eye and put names to them. Then look at the book (covering the names with a piece of paper) and try to recall all the names. If you remember all the names and faces after just two minutes, well done! If you can't do this in that time, try again

for another two minutes, and another. At this stage, accuracy is more important than speed. Now give yourself a break and try again 24 hours later. If you can still remember all the names and faces, you're doing really well.

Arthur
Penrose

Susie
Adder

Michael
Brown

Tim
Strawton

Alice
Short

Maggi
Clayton

Your score:

REVISION TASK 6

Dates

(Pages 84–85)

Suggested revision: See how much of your timeline you can still draw from memory. Take a look at the original and fill in any gaps.

The test

1 In which year was Alfred Nobel born?
2 What happened in Orlando, Florida in 1971?
3 When did Herschel discover Uranus has two moons?
4 When did Iceland become an independent republic?
5 When did Lincoln announce the end of slavery?
6 When was Trotsky expelled from the Communist Party?
7 When did the author of the Tarzan books die?
8 When was the province of Quebec founded?
9 When was Sigourney Weaver born?
10 When was Juan Peron born?

Each correct answer   **5 points**

REVISION TASK 7

Shopping list

(Pages 86–87)

Suggested revision: You can take a very quick look at the original list on page 87. With luck, you have adapted this by now and it has become your own shopping list (in which case you might be better off not completing this test as it might confuse you).

The test

Simply write down the whole list from memory and check your answers against the original.

Each correct item   **2 points**

Your score:

Your score:

REVISION TASK 8
Signs of the zodiac

(Pages 88–89)

Suggested revision: Remember to use both visual and listening cues for this task. Close your eyes and visualize your zodiac diagram, then recite all the signs and their dates in order.

The test

1 Which sign comes after Virgo?
2 Which sign comes before Gemini?
3 Name the Water signs.
4 Is Libra a Fire sign?
5 Which sign covers most of August?
6 Which sign covers January and part of February?
7 Which sign is represented by a pair of scales?
8 Which sign are you born under if your birthday is 15 May?
9 A December baby is most likely to be born under which sign?
10 Name one sign from each of Water, Earth and Fire.

Each correct answer   **5 points**

REVISION TASK 9
Animal farm

(Pages 90–91)

Suggested revision: Spend a few minutes revisiting the pictures. Remember to read out loud the names of the animals and touch them as you do so. Close your eyes and try to visualize the whole set of pictures in your mind's eye.

The test

1 What is to the right of the cow?
2 Where is the tiger?
3 Are the sheep above or below the porcupine?
4 Where is the grizzly bear in relation to the polar bear?
5 Where is the leopard?
6 Is the panda to the left or the right of the giraffes?
7 Where is the lion in relation to the fox?
8 Is there a cobra in the picture?
9 Is there an orang-utan in the picture?
10 Where is the elephant in relation to the ostrich?

Each correct answer   **5 points**

Your score:

Your score:

REVISION TASK 10

Kings and queens of England

(Pages 92–93)

Suggested revision: Make sure you have the mnemonic off pat and know what it means. Spend some time going over the pages and use both visual and verbal clues to try to fix the names in your memory.

The test

1 Who lost his jewels in The Wash?
2 How many Edwards are there?
3 Which monarch was the victor of Agincourt?
4 Who succeeded Henry II?
5 What events separate the House of Lancaster and the House of York?
6 Who came before and after Elizabeth I?
7 Who came after Richard III?
8 Who came after the three Neds?
9 Who came before Victoria?
10 Who was Elizabeth II's grandfather?

Each correct answer   **5 points**

REVISION TASK 11

Café Olé

(Pages 94–95)

Suggested revision: This was a tough exercise the first time around and, now that some time has elapsed, you may well find it even tougher. Don't panic! Relax and let the memory you created earlier come back to you. If you have made a point of memorizing something it will still be there, and all you need do is encourage it to surface.

The test

1 Who had the croissant?
2 Who ate the English breakfast?
3 What went with the slice of fruit cake?
4 Who had the cherry pie?
5 What did the customer drink with his pepperoni pizza?
6 Who had the fried chicken?
7 Who drank soda water?
8 Who had sausage and beans?
9 Who liked honey?
10 Who had the raisin scone?

Each correct answer   **5 points**

Your score:

Your score:

REVISION TASK 12
Ticket to ride

(Pages 96–97)

Suggested revision: This was a tough test, so it makes sense to take time going over it again. Of course, if you've been super diligent, you will have included this test in your regular reviews, but it is likely that you've let it lapse. So spend time now reading it out loud, and looking it over to re-energize your visual memory. When you read the lists of places, use a silly voice of some sort. A rhythm or a song tune will work wonders. If any of the place names have odd associations for you, don't hesitate to make a note of that. Remember to keep it stupid, childish and even vulgar because these are the things that stick in the mind.

The test

1 Which platform does the Thorpe train leave from?
2 Which line is Abbey Morton on?
3 Which train is delayed and by how long?
4 Which train has been cancelled?
5 Which platform has trains to Gromby?
6 When is the Dudstead train supposed to arrive?
7 Which line is Carlton on?
8 Which station precedes Dewenter?
9 Which station precedes Harling?
10 What time does the Fairfield train depart?

Each correct answer   **5 points**

Your score:

REVISION TASK 13
Presidents of the USA

(Pages 98–101)

Suggested revision: There is really no substitute for splitting the list into small blocks and learning them to a rhythm. Try to get the pictures fixed in your mind. They will provide valuable cues. Use silly associations wherever possible – want to remember Garfield? Think of the cartoon cat! Get all the well-known presidents lodged in your memory (if you forget Washington, Lincoln or Kennedy, there is really no hope for you). Once you have a framework, you can start to fill in the gaps. Can you do them out of order? Let's see.

The test

1 Who came between Lincoln and Grant?
2 Who came after Teddy Roosevelt?
3 Who came before Eisenhower?
4 What are the initials of the first President Bush?
5 Who came before Garfield?
6 Who did Hoover succeed?
7 Who came before and after Nixon?
8 Who preceded Reagan?
9 Who came before Harry Truman?
10 Who came after Andrew Jackson?

Each correct answer   **5 points**

Your score:

REVISION TASK 14

Learning Braille

(Pages 102–103)

Suggested revision: Get out your homemade Braille cards and refresh your memory. Remember, sighted people should learn Braille by sight as well as touch. There's no point in not using all the tools at your disposal. You might,

however, like to test your reading speed by working with your eyes shut. Apparently, experienced Braille users can read almost as fast as a sighted person. Give it a try and see how you get on. Now try to read the following by sight.

The test

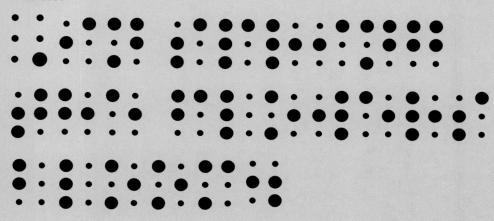

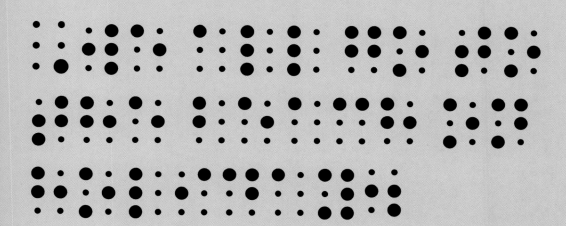

Each correct answer   **5 points**

Your score:

Check your answers on page 157.

REVISION TASK 15

Wine bottle sizes and names

(Pages 104–105)

Suggested revision: The pictures should give you all the information you need and, luckily, because bottle names are all 'odd' words, they are very memorable. The hard bit is working out the variations for champagne, Bordeaux and Burgundy. Write down all you can remember (making a table just like the one we printed), and then add bits as you can. Work in pencil so you can correct mistakes.

The test

1　What is a triple-sized bottle of Bordeaux called?
2　What is a double-sized bottle of any wine called?
3　How many bottles make a Methuselah?
4　Which bottle of Bordeaux represents 6 normal bottles?
5　What is the largest bottle of wine you can get?
6　How many normal bottles are in a Balthazar?
7　How many normal bottles are in a Double Magnum?
8　What is a Picolo?
9　What is a Nebuchadnezzar?
10　What is an Imperial?

Each correct answer　　　　　**5 points**

For **5 extra points** add the missing information to the illustration below

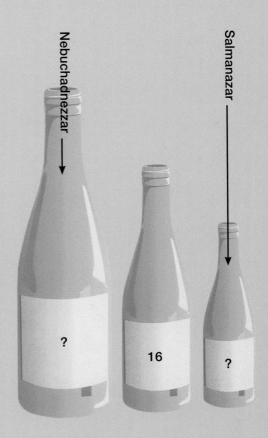

Your score:

REVISION TASK 16
Beaufort Scale

(Pages 106–107)

Suggested revision: Make a point of noticing the wind speed each day and working out its likely rating on the Beaufort Scale. This will take care of the lower wind speeds, though you may have to wait for a while to experience the higher ones. Read through the description of the scale one more time and then try to answer the following questions.

The test

1 What does smoke do in a Force 1 wind?
2 What force is required to set large branches in motion?
3 What force constitutes a gale?
4 What is another name for Force 12?
5 What effect does a Force 3 have on trees?
6 What force is also known as Violent Storm?
7 What wind force is the first to make using an umbrella difficult?
8 What grades come between Calm and Fresh Breeze?
9 At what force would you observe whole trees in motion?
10 At what force would slight structural damage occur?

Each correct answer   **5 points**

REVISION TASK 17
Roman numerals

(Page 108)

Suggested revision: As long as you understand the system, you should be able to do Roman numerals by now without revision. If you don't understand the system, you need to brush up on the rules and remind yourself of the meanings of the more unusual letters (everyone remembers I, V, X, C and M, but many people get caught out on D and L). Also, remind yourself about letters with an overscore being multiplied by 1,000 – it does make quite a difference if you forget!

The test

Put the following into Roman numerals:

1 128
2 436
3 1300
4 21
5 2345

What do these numerals stand for?

1 XXIV
2 MCVII
3 CXVII
4 MDCXVI
5 DLV

See page 157 for the answers.

Each correct answer   **5 points**

Your score:

Your score:

REVISION TASK 18

Memorizing unusual capital cities

(Pages 109–111)

Suggested revision: If you followed the advice given earlier you should have a comprehensive knowledge of world geography. Use any silly, childish or weird sounding associations you can to get names to stick in your mind. Weird names work best! Can you ever forget Burkina Faso's capital Ouagadougou?

The test

1 What is the capital of Ecuador?
2 What is the capital of Morocco?
3 Paramaribo is the capital of which country?
4 Where would you find Muscat?
5 What is the capital of Qatar?
6 Of which country is Asmara the capital?
7 What is the capital of Grenada?
8 Where would you find Vientiane?
9 Of which country is Libreville the capital?
10 Where would you find Tegucigalpa?

Each correct answer   **5 points**

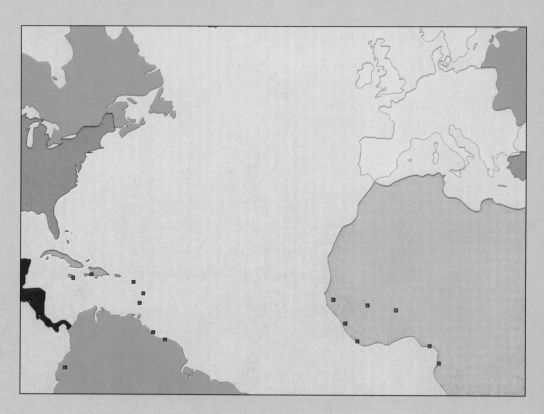

As an extra test of your skills, see how many of the cities in the map above you can identify correctly.

Your score:

REVISION TASK 19

Memorizing cloud types

(Pages 112–113)

Suggested revision: If you have made a habit of observing cloud types, you should have the whole system well memorized by now. Because you can watch a free 'cloud show' outside your window each day, the whole cloud system should make perfect sense (and your powers of weather prediction will also increase).

The test

1 Which clouds do you find in a 'mackerel sky'?
2 Which cloud produces a halo effect?
3 What does 'cumulus' mean?
4 What does 'cirrus' mean?
5 Does 'nimbus' mean the same as 'snow'?
6 Which clouds do you associate with a bright, sunny day?
7 Which form of cloud is only found at the lowest level?
8 Which is the highest cloud form?
9 What does 'stratus' mean?
10 Identify the cloud types shown here.

Each correct answer   **5 points**

Your score:

REVISION TASK 20

Learn semaphore

(Pages 114–117)

Suggested revision: Quickly run through the whole system. Don't just read about it, do it! The 'learning by doing' method is very important here.

The test

Signal the following (get someone to read out the questions and check your signalling against the alphabet on page 115).

1 It was a fine and a pleasant day.
2 Flowers regularly bloom in spring.
3 My two sons are called Fred and Charlie.
4 I saw two zebras and a tiger at the zoo.
5 Signalling gets tiring after a very short time.

Start with **50 points** and deduct **5 points** for each error. For an extra **10 points**, work out the sentence signalled below.

See page 157 for the answer.

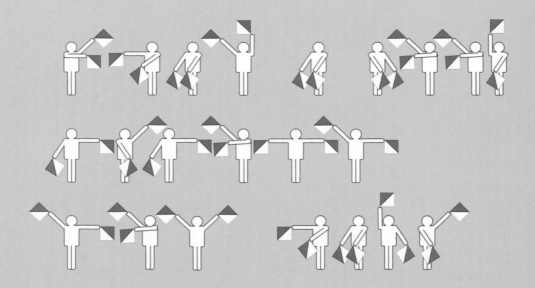

Your score:

REVISION TASK 21

Learn Morse code

(Pages 118–119)

Suggested revision: Tap your way through the alphabet a couple of times. If you memorized this code properly the first time around, you shouldn't need to look at it now.

The test

Tap out the following messages. Get someone to check you. Go for accuracy rather than speed.

1 They do not sell chocolate at the corner shop.
2 Dogs are a nuisance when they bark at night.
3 Cauliflower goes well with ham.
4 I like to work in the garden every day in summer.
5 On winter evenings I like to gaze at the stars.
6 I hope to go on holiday to Zanzibar.
7 My mother needs an x-ray on her hip.
8 I bought a yacht and painted it green.
9 Let's all go out for dinner together.
10 Morse code is enough to make you dash your head against a wall.

Each correct answer   **5 points**

REVISION TASK 22

Memorize something really confusing

(Pages 120–121)

The test

1 What colour is APPLE?
2 Where is SILVER?
3 What colour is SKY?
4 What is two places to the right of PURPLE?
5 What is two places up from BROWN?
6 Where is BLUE?
7 What colour is COAL?
8 What is at the top of the third column?
9 What colour is GOLD?
10 Where is ORANGE?

Each correct answer   **5 points**

Your score:

Your score:

REVISION TASK 23
Comprehension

(Pages 122–123)

Suggested revision: If you learnt this piece thoroughly the first time you tried it, you may well find that much of it has stuck with you. A few minutes spent re-reading the piece should be all you need to bring the memory back into sharp focus. Some people find it helpful to think of real people with the same names as the characters in the story. If you don't happen to have friends and relations with the right names, you can always borrow celebrities and work them into your drama.

The test

1 Who used to go out with Laura?
2 What meat does Mark dislike?
3 Who comes from Wales?
4 Where does Sophie work?
5 Where is the Maharajah?
6 When did Pete and Laura get engaged?
7 What is Laura unable to eat?
8 Where is the cinema?
9 Who loves Mark?
10 What does Sinead do for a living?

Each correct answer   **5 points**

REVISION TASK 24
Memorize a table of symbols

(Pages 124–125)

Suggested revision: Take a few minutes to refresh your visualization of the table. Try to draw it from memory. When you are satisfied that you have it fixed in your mind's eye, test yourself with the following questions.

The test

1 Which symbol is at the top of the right hand column?
2 What comes immediately below ‡ ?
3 What is to the right of ✳ ?
4 What is two places below ± ?
5 What is at the far end of the row that starts with ✿ ?
6 What is at the bottom of the column that starts with ✻ ?
7 What is at the beginning of the row that ends with Ω ?
8 What is directly above # ?
9 Can you remember all the symbols that surround ‡ ?
10 Where is ≈ ?

Each correct answer   **5 points**

Your score:

Your score:

REVISION TASK 25
Learning to tie knots

(Pages 126–127)

Suggested revision: The type of memory you acquire by feel is extraordinarily tenacious, so you shouldn't need to revise for this test.

The test
Tie each of these knots.

Jug sling

Surgeon's knot

True lover's knot

Shamrock knot

Blood bight

10 points for each knot that matches exactly the pictures on pages 126–129.

REVISION TASK 26
Learning long words

(Pages 130–131)

Suggested revision: Take a look at each word ONCE ONLY. That should be enough to bring them to mind again.

The test
Get someone to read out the words, one at a time, and try to write them down from memory.

Honorificabilitudinity
Dihydroxylphenylalanine
Gynotikolobomassophile
Hexamethylenetetramine
Bathysiderodromophobia
Rhombicosidodecahedron
Pseudomonocotyledonous
Hippopotomonstrosesquippedaliophobia
Hepaticocholangiocholecystenterostomies
Pneumonoultramicroscopicsilicovoicanoconiosis
Aequeosalinocalcalinosetaceoaluminosocupreovitriolic
Osseocarnisanguineoviscericartilagninonervomedullary

Start with **50 points** and then deduct **1 point** for each mistake. Get someone to check your efforts against the book.

Your score:

Your score:

REVISION TASK 27

Learn the battles of the American Civil War

(Pages 132–133)

Suggested revision: This was one of the toughest tests in the book so, if you still do not achieve 100 per cent, don't get too disheartened. Try writing out a list from memory and then work on filling in the gaps. This is one of those tasks that is very hard to accomplish unless you have at least some understanding of the subject. If you looked up a potted history of the war earlier your efforts should have borne more fruit than if you merely tried to learn the facts in isolation.

The test

1 What year was the Battle of Cold Harbor?
2 Which battle took place in Tennessee in 1863?
3 By what other name are the two battles of Manasses known?
4 Where is Antietam Creek?
5 In which year was the Battle of Seven Days?
6 What was the last battle of the war?
7 What was the first battle of the war?
8 When was the siege of Petersburg?
9 When was the Battle of Chickamauga?
10 When was the Battle of Shiloh?

Each correct answer   **5 points**

Your score:

REVISION TASK 28

The Periodic Table of elements

(Pages 134–135)

Suggested revision: This was a brutally hard task and, if you completed it, you should congratulate yourself. If you really memorized the whole table it will have stayed with you and you will need only a swift rehearsal to get all the questions right. If, however, you skimped on the work before, nothing is going to save you now.

The test

1 What does Ti stand for?
2 What is the symbol for molybdenum?
3 What comes directly below hydrogen?
4 What comes just below sodium?
5 What does Y stand for?
6 What comes after zirconium?
7 What does Rf stand for?
8 What is the symbol for magnesium?
9 What does the symbol Uuq stand for?
10 What does Sb stand for?

Each correct answer   **5 points**

Your score:

REVISION TASK 29

Learn some basic Chinese characters

(pages 136–137)

Suggested revision: This should be an easy task as long as you remembered the clues that were given about each character. A quick glance should bring it all back to mind.

The test

Identify the following characters:

山 女 門
車 馬 心
耳 齒 酉 肉

Each correct answer   **5 points**

Your score:

Answers

Roman numerals (page 108)

XV	XXXV
CCXXXIX	CDXXVI
V̄CCXLIV	V̄MMDCCCXC
V̄LDCCCLIX	

Learn semaphore (pages 116–117)

1 Reading semaphore is easy with practice.
2 The meeting place has changed.
3 We are landing at midnight.
4 My speed of translation improves all the time.

Braille (page 147)

1 In spring the flowers bloom.
2 We all go to the beach on holiday.

Roman numerals (revision – page 149)

Converting into Roman numerals:
1 CXXVIII
2 CDXXXVI
3 MCCC
4 XXI
5 MMCCCXLV

Converting into numerals:
1 24
2 1107
3 117
4 1616
5 555

Learn semaphore (revision – page 152)

What a good memory you have.

Index

Acknowledgements

I should like to thank my wife, Doris, and my kids, Alex and Gina, for the help, ideas and encouragement they contributed during the writing of this book. I'd also like to thank all the people who took part in my memory seminars and provided me with guinea pigs on whom to test my ideas.

Picture credits

The publisher wishes to thank the organizations listed below for their kind permission to reproduce the photographs in this book. Every effort has been made to acknowledge the pictures, however we apologize if there are any unintentional omissions.

B = bottom; L= left; R = right; T = top; C = centre.

ARS-USDA /91.
Clip Art / 99, 100, 101, 110, 111.
Digital Stock /16, 54CL.
Digital Vision / 15, 16,17T, 20CL, 20C, 20n, 20TR, 20T, 21, 22, 27, 29, 30, 44, 45, 55CR, 58, 86, 87, 91, 108.
Illustrated London News /92, 132.
Photo Disc / 14, 20BR, 20B, 21, 54BL, 54B, 55CL.
Stockbyte / 17B, 21, 54TR, 54BR, 55B, 86, 87.
US Fish & Wildlife Service /91.

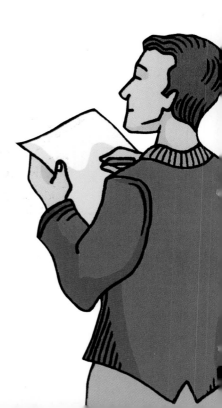